Self Assessment Questio

Yousaf Ali

Self Assessment Questions in Rheumatology

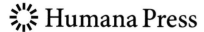 Humana Press

Yousaf Ali MD, FACR
Assistant Clinical Professor of Medicine
Brown University
Rhode Island
Yousafali1@gmail.com

ISBN: 978-1-934115-52-7   e-ISBN: 978-1-59745-497-1
DOI: 10.1007/978-1-59745-497-1

Library of Congress Control Number: 2008942270

springer.com

Preface

This book is for postgraduate fellows, internists, and students interested in rheumatology. It contains real cases and is designed to stimulate thought and further reading in this rapidly evolving specialty.

I have included a series of common and uncommon cases that I have seen over the past decade in a busy consultative practice and have inserted up-to-date references and questions you may be asked on ward rounds or in clinic. My hope is that it will be a useful adjunct for physicians preparing for examinations or entering the field and will stimulate further interest.

I would like to acknowledge my mentors Pierre Bouloux, MD, Tom Cooney, MD and thank Atul Deodhar, MD for his careful review of the manuscript.

This book is dedicated to my parents and wife Batool who have made many sacrifices for which I remain eternally grateful.

Brooklyn, NY

Yousaf Ali

Contents

Question 1

A 56-year-old female presents with arthralgias and fatigue. Lab work is unremarkable apart from normocytic anemia and Howell Jolly bodies on peripheral smear. Her examination reveals a blistering rash on the elbows.

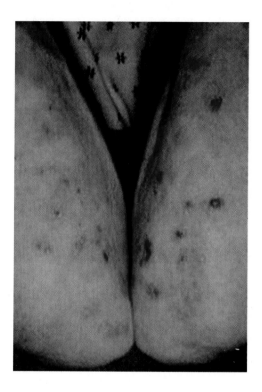

What is the most likely diagnosis?
What are the other hematologic complications of this disease?

Yousaf Ali, *Self Assessment Questions in Rheumatology,* DOI: 10.1007/ 978-1-59745-497-1,
Humana Press, a part of Springer Science + Business Media, LLC 2009

Answer: Celiac disease (CD)

This disease is more common in Northern European ancestry characterized by sensitivity to gluten. Patients present with symptoms of malabsorption, arthralgia, skin rash, and hematologic disorders. Dermatitis herpeteformis is a blistering skin rash seen in this condition. Howell Jolly bodies reflect nuclear remnants that persist due to hyposplenism. Hematologic complications of CD include anemia due to malabsorption of iron, B12, or folate; lymphoma, leucopenia, thromboembolism, and IgA deficiency.

Halfdanarson TR, Litzow MR, Murray JA. Hematologic manifestations of celiac disease. Blood. 2007 Jan 15;109(2):412–21.

Question 2

A 35-year-old female is referred for evaluation of + antinuclear antibodies (ANA). She is asymptomatic. Her lab work reveals ANA 1:320 homogeneous pattern; extractable nuclear antigens are negative. Hematologic and renal function values are normal and urinalysis is without sediment. Her examination is unremarkable apart from a smooth nontender goiter. The past medical history is significant for Hashimoto's thyroiditis. No rash, synovitis, or serositis is observed.

What is the most likely diagnosis?
What further treatment or investigations are warranted?

Yousaf Ali, *Self Assessment Questions in Rheumatology,* DOI: 10.1007/ 978-1-59745-497-1,
Humana Press, a part of Springer Science + Business Media, LLC 2009

Answer: Hashimotos thyroiditis

The ANA is most likely of no clinical significance. Up to 46% of patients with autoimmune thyroid disease have positive antinuclear antibodies. Assuming that the patient remains asymptomatic no further intervention is warranted.

Petri M, Karlson EW, Cooper DS, Ladenson PW. Autoantibody tests in autoimmune thyroid disease: a case-control study. J Rheumatol. 1991 Oct;18(10):1529–31.

Question 3

You are asked to evaluate a 74-year-old male with joint pain. He was recently admitted after a bout of diverticulitis. On examination he has polyarticular synovitis, and arthrocentesis reveals multiple intracellular uric acid (UA) crystals diagnostic of gout. Lab values: UA = 5.5 mg/dl, WBC = 10.5, HB = 11.5, Plts = 550, and creatinine = 2.8 mg/dl.

How would you best manage this patient's gout? Why is the uric acid normal?

Yousaf Ali, *Self Assessment Questions in Rheumatology,* DOI: 10.1007/ 978-1-59745-497-1,
Humana Press, a part of Springer Science + Business Media, LLC 2009

Answer: Oral corticosteroids

This is a common inpatient scenario. A stable patient with renal failure is admitted and undergoes a stressful procedure that triggers gout. Treatment of acute gout involves high-dose NSAID, colchicine, or corticosteroids. In a patient with renal failure and diverticular inflammation, NSAIDs and colchicine should be avoided since they are poorly tolerated. A monoarticular presentation could be injected with local intraarticular corticosteroid assuming that the cultures are negative. In this patient with polyarticular gout a short burst of oral corticosteroid is the best option.

Uric acid levels fall and are often normal during an attack and should not be used as a diagnostic test.

Terkeltaub RA. Clinical practice. Gout. N Engl J Med. 2003 Oct 23;349(17):1647–55.

The best drug for acute gout in pt. c̄ renal disease

= Steroids

Question 4

A 55-year-old female with longstanding Sjogrens syndrome (SS) presents with new onset of lethargy, hypokalemia, and nephrocalcinosis. Her metabolic profile reveals an anion gap metabolic acidosis, hypokalemia, and alkaline urine. A skeletal survey reveals diffuse osteopenia.

What complication has occurred?

Yousaf Ali, *Self Assessment Questions in Rheumatology*, DOI: 10.1007/ 978-1-59745-497-1,
Humana Press, a part of Springer Science + Business Media, LLC 2009

Answer: Distal type 1 renal tubular acidosis (RTA)

This is a rare but important complication of SS. Distal RTA occurs due to failure to acidify urine to a pH < 5.3. This results in anion gap acidosis, hypokalemia, nephrocalcinosis, and bone demineralization. The lymphocytes that invade the tubular epithelial cells are CD8-positive, i.e., cytotoxic T cells and similar to those found in the salivary glands of patients with Sjögren's syndrome. The same immunological process is probably operative in the renal tubulointerstitial tissue as in the salivary glands to induce the characteristic tissue changes of Sjögren's syndrome.

Matsumura R, Kondo Y, Sugiyama T, Sueishi M, Koike T, Takabayashi K, Tomioka H, Yoshida S, Tsuchida H. Immunohistochemical identification of infiltrating mononuclear cells in tubulointerstitial nephritis associated with Sjögren's syndrome. Clin Nephrol. 1988 Dec;30(6):335–40.

Moutsopoulos HM, Cledes J, Skopouli FN, Elisaf M, Youinou P. Nephrocalcinosis in Sjögren's syndrome: a late sequela of renal tubular acidosis. J Intern Med. 1991 Aug;230(2):187–91.

Wrong OM. Immune-related potassium-losing interstitial nephritis: a comparison with distal renal tubular acidosis. QJM 1993;86(8):513–42.

Question 5

A 47-year-old patient with Crohn's disease presents for evaluation of new onset arthritis. She has a 20-year history of colitis managed with sulfasalazine and local corticosteroid suppositories. Infliximab at 5 mg/kg was recently commenced due to persistent disease activity. She arrives with new onset polyarticular joint pain. On examination she has synovitis of the small joints of the hands and a warm knee effusion. Lab work: WBC = 2.8, Hb = 11.2 g/dl, platelets = 554, ESR = 66, ANA = 1:640, RF = 54, and renal and liver studies normal.

What is the most likely diagnosis?
What further tests can confirm this?
How would you manage this patient?

Yousaf Ali, *Self Assessment Questions in Rheumatology,* DOI: 10.1007/ 978-1-59745-497-1,
Humana Press, a part of Springer Science+Business Media, LLC 2009

Answer: Infliximab-induced SLE

This patient presents with a new polyarticular flare after commencing infliximab. The differential diagnosis is between Crohn's related arthropathy and drug-induced SLE. The latter is more likely given the leucopenia and +ANA. Infliximab has been reported to induce antinuclear antibodies and can cause drug-induced SLE. Prompt discontinuation of the drug is warranted. Further testing includes checking antibodies to histone protein, extractable nuclear antigens, serum complements, differential cell count to look for lymphopenia, and renal function. Typically drug-induced SLE does not involve major organ systems.

Watts RA. Musculoskeletal and systemic reactions to biological therapeutic agents. Curr Opin Rheumatol. 2000 Jan;12(1):49–52.

Question 6

A 67-year-old man presents with left groin pain. His internist has ordered a bone scan and radiograph, which he would like you to interpret. The hip radiograph reveals stage 4 osteoarthritis (OA). Fig. 1 shows the bone scan.

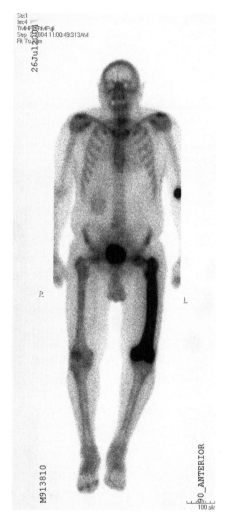

Fig. 1

What is the most likely diagnosis?
How would you best manage this patient's bone pain?
What complications may occur?

Yousaf Ali, *Self Assessment Questions in Rheumatology,* DOI: 10.1007/ 978-1-59745-497-1,
Humana Press, a part of Springer Science + Business Media, LLC 2009

Answer: Paget's disease

This bone scan shows tibial bowing and marked uptake in the left femur consistent with Paget's disease. The bone pain should be managed by oral or intravenous bisphosphonates. Zoledronic acid was approved in the USA in 2007 as a single, once annual intravenous infusion for the treatment of Paget's disease. Complications of Paget's disease include fracture, high-output heart failure, deafness, and, very rarely, osteosarcoma.

Bone HG. Nonmalignant complications of Paget's disease. J Bone Miner Res. 2006 Dec;21 Suppl 2:P64–P68. Review.

Keating GM, Scott LJ. Zoledronic acid: a review of its use in the treatment of Paget's disease of bone. Drugs. 2007;67(5):793–804.

Question 7

A 45-year-old female with 5 years of rheumatoid arthritis (RA) presents with increasing pain and stiffness. On examination she has synovitis of the mcp and pip joints with associated joint tenderness. Her current regimen includes plaquenil 200 mg twice daily, sulfasalazine 3 g daily, and folate. Labs reveal ESR = 25 mm/h, +RF, +CCP antibody. CRP is 162 mg/l and disease activity score (DAS) is high. Radiographs reveal periarticular erosions.

What is the significance of the +CCP antibody?
How would you manage her RA?

Yousaf Ali, *Self Assessment Questions in Rheumatology,* DOI: 10.1007/ 978-1-59745-497-1,
Humana Press, a part of Springer Science + Business Media, LLC 2009

Answer: The CCP antibody predicts disease severity and progression to erosions. Methotrexate should be added

She has aggressive erosive disease with elevated markers of inflammation and high-titer CCP antibody. Since she is actively symptomatic despite two disease-modifying antirheumatic drugs (DMARDs) it is time to add methotrexate (MTX). Triple therapy is superior to single agents although there are many pills to take weekly. A short bridge of corticosteroids may also be helpful in decreasing inflammatory symptoms. Some rheumatologists will argue that aggressive early use of tumor necrosis factor (TNF) antagonists is also indicated. Since these are expensive medications and the patient has not failed the "gold standard" they should be reserved unless she fails to respond to MTX. This algorithm may change as cost–benefit data on the existing agents become available and as newer, safer, and more efficacious agents are introduced.

O'Dell JR, Leff R, Paulsen G, Haire C, Mallek J, Eckhoff PJ, Fernandez A, Blakely K, Wees S, Stoner J, Hadley S, Felt J, Palmer W, Waytz P, Churchill M, Klassen L, Moore G. Treatment of rheumatoid arthritis with methotrexate and hydroxychloroquine, methotrexate and sulfasalazine, or a combination of the three medications: results of a two-year, randomized, double-blind, placebo-controlled trial. Arthritis Rheum. 2002 May;46(5):1164–70.

Question 8

A 68-year-old female is referred for diffuse joint pain and fatigue of 2 years duration. Her PMH is consistent with depression, posttraumatic stress disorder (PTSD), and hypothyroidism. Hematologic, biochemical, and immunologic studies are negative. Inflammatory markers are not elevated. On examination she has palatal hypertrophy and is markedly obese. Cardiac examination reveals a loud S2 with RV heave. Pulmonary examination is normal. She has pitting edema and multiple tender points to palpation but no synovitis.

What is the most likely diagnosis?
What investigations, if any, are appropriate?
How would you manage her?

Yousaf Ali, *Self Assessment Questions in Rheumatology,* DOI: 10.1007/ 978-1-59745-497-1,
Humana Press, a part of Springer Science + Business Media, LLC 2009

Answer: Obstructive sleep apnea with pulmonary hypertension and benign arthralgias/fibromyalgia

Patients with chronic sleep apnea develop pulmonary hypertension due to hypoxemia and develop subsequent right-sided pulmonary hypertension. A distinct relationship exists between poor sleep quality and pain intensity. This patient most likely has fibromyalgia, which is characterized by widespread pain, insomnia, and tender points. Investigations should focus around excluding an organic cause for pain, managing sleep disturbance, and treating underlying sleep apnea and depression. Physical therapy, counseling, and aerobic exercise have also been found to be useful.

Clauw DJ. Fibromyalgia: update on mechanisms and management. J Clin Rheumatol. 2007 Apr; 13(2):102–9.

Question 9

A 74-year-old male with chronic erosive RA of 35 years duration presents with new onset bipedal edema. Current treatment regimen includes low-dose MTX, and 5-mg prednisone. His labs reveal Hb = 10.8, MCV = 88, and platelets = 544. Creatinine is 0.8 mg/dl. ESR = 67 mm/h. Cardiac and pulmonary examinations are normal. An ECHO reveals increased left ventricular wall thickness, abnormal myocardial reflectivity, and a small pericardial effusion pattern.

What is the most likely diagnosis?
What further tests are warranted?
How would you manage him?

Yousaf Ali, *Self Assessment Questions in Rheumatology,* DOI: 10.1007/ 978-1-59745-497-1,
Humana Press, a part of Springer Science + Business Media, LLC 2009

Answer: This patient has developed secondary amyloidosis due to chronic inflammation

Amyloidosis is a systemic disease characterized by deposition of insoluble beta pleated sheets of protein in various organs. The diagnosis can be confirmed by congo red staining of subcutaneous fat. Although it is primary amyloidosis that usually affects the myocardium it can also occur with the secondary form. His lower extremity edema might be explained by heart failure but nephrotic syndrome also needs to be excluded. Treatment of secondary amyloidosis is often unsatisfactory and primarily involves treatment of the underlying disease.

Aresté JF, Solé JMN, Vaquero CG, García JV, Escofet DR. Secondary amyloidosis in rheumatoid arthritis. A clinical study of 29 patients. Ann Med Intern. 1999 Dec;16(12):6.

Voskuyl AE. The heart and cardiovascular manifestations in rheumatoid arthritis. Rheumatology. 2006 Oct;45 Suppl 4:iv4–iv7. Review.

Question 10

A 25-year-old female with a 5-year history of SLE presents with increasing edema of 1-week duration. Her medications include hydroxychloroquine 200 mg twice daily. She has a history of cervical intraepithelial neoplasia and human papilloma virus (HPV). Lab data reveal Hb = 10.5, WBC = 3.2, and creatinine = 0.6 mg/dl. Urinalysis shows 4+ proteinuria, red cell casts, and active sediment. A renal biopsy shows active glomerulonephritis with full-house immunofluorescence interpreted as stage IV active diffuse proliferative glomerulonephritis (DPGN).

How would you manage this condition?

Yousaf Ali, *Self Assessment Questions in Rheumatology,* DOI: 10.1007/ 978-1-59745-497-1,
Humana Press, a part of Springer Science+Business Media, LLC 2009

Answer: Treat with mycophenylate mofetil

This patient has class IV lupus nephritis, which, untreated, has a high risk of progression to chronic renal failure. The standard of care has been pulse dose methylprednisolone with intravenous cyclophosphamide given initially as monthly pulses and subsequently quarterly for a 2-year period. Patients with SLE who have received IV cytoxan have a higher risk of progression to cervical dysplasia, and therefore in this patient mycophenylate mofetil is a better alternative with equal efficacy and less toxicity.

Bateman H, Yazici Y, Leff L, Peterson M, Paget SA. Increased cervical dysplasia in intravenous cyclophosphamide-treated patients with SLE: a preliminary study. Lupus. 2000;9(7):542–4.

Ginzler EM, Dooley MA, Aranow C, Kim MY, Buyon J, Merrill JT, Petri M, Gilkeson GS, Wallace DJ, Weisman MH, Appel GB. Mycophenolate mofetil or intravenous cyclophosphamide for lupus nephritis. N Engl J Med. 2005 Nov 24;353(21):2219–28.

Ognenovski VM, Marder W, Somers EC, Johnston CM, Farrehi JG, Selvaggi SM, McCune WJ. Increased incidence of cervical intraepithelial neoplasia in women with systemic lupus erythematosus treated with intravenous cyclophosphamide. J Rheumatol. 2004 Sep;31(9):1763–7.

Question 11

A 66-year-old male was seen with a history of recurrent oral ulceration. He has no other symptoms. PMH includes posterior uveitis and aseptic meningitis. On examination he has painful eythematous lesions on the anterior shins. Labs reveal a mild normocytic anemia.

What is the most likely diagnosis?

Yousaf Ali, *Self Assessment Questions in Rheumatology,* DOI: 10.1007/ 978-1-59745-497-1,
Humana Press, a part of Springer Science + Business Media, LLC 2009

Answer: Behcet's syndrome complicated by erythema nodosum

This is a condition more commonly seen in people who live on the Silk route from the Mediterranean basin to China. There is a strong association with HLA B51. The disease is characterized by thrombophlebitis, recurrent orogenital apthous ulceration, posterior uveitis, and meningoencephalitis. Cutaneous findings include a positive pathergy test, pseudofolliculitis, or erythema nodosum. Rarely pulmonary artery aneurysms can occur.

Sakane T, Takeno M, Suzuki N, Inaba G. Behcet's disease. N Engl J Med. 1999 Oct 21;341(17):1284–91.

Question 12

A 19-year-old female with SLE consults you for contraceptive advice. She is sexually active and has a history of serositis, leucopenia, and arthritis. Current medications include azathioprine 100 mg/daily and naprosyn 500 mg twice daily. Labs: WBC = 2.4, Hb = 10.5, platelets = 125,000, lupus anticoagulant present, PTT = 55 s, and anticardiolipin (ACA) antibody IgM/IgG strongly positive.

What advice would you give her regarding contraception?

Yousaf Ali, *Self Assessment Questions in Rheumatology,* DOI: 10.1007/ 978-1-59745-497-1,
Humana Press, a part of Springer Science+Business Media, LLC 2009

Answer: She should be advised to use barrier protection, progesterone only pill or IUCD's

This patient has a prolonged partial thromboplastin time, thrombocytopenia, strongly positive ACA's, and circulating lupus anticoagulant. Although the patient has not had prior thromboses she is at high risk for developing antiphospholipid antibody syndrome in view of these blood tests. These patients are hypercoagulable and should not be given estrogen-containing products due to the increased risk of thrombosis. She should be advised to use barrier protection, progesterone-only pill, or IUCDs. ACOG recommends that in SLE, estrogen-containing contraceptives be avoided in patients with vascular disease, nephritis, or ACA.

ACOG Committee on Practice Bulletins. Gynecology. ACOG Practice Bulletin No. 73: Use of hormonal contraception in women with coexisting medical conditions. Obstet Gynecol. 2006 Jun;107(6):1453–72.

Lakasing L, Khamashta M. Contraceptive practices in women with systemic lupus erythematosus and/or antiphospholipid syndrome: what advice should we be giving? J Fam Plann Reprod Health Care. 2001 Jan;27(1):7–12.

Question 13

A 23-year-old female has new onset edema following a course of high-dose steroids for poison ivy. On examination BP = 166/110, loud S2, and clear lungs without jugular distension. She has abnormal nail fold capillary examination with dilated loops and dropout. There is no sclerodactly, malar rash, synovitis, or weakness. Urinalysis shows nephritic range proteinuria with no cellular casts. ANA is 1:10250, normal complements, negative centromere/ Scl-70/ANCA antibodies. Platelets 75 k, +schistocytes on peripheral smear.

What is the most likely diagnosis?

Yousaf Ali, *Self Assessment Questions in Rheumatology,* DOI: 10.1007/ 978-1-59745-497-1,
Humana Press, a part of Springer Science+Business Media, LLC 2009

Answer: SRC sine scleroderma

This patient most likely has scleroderma renal crisis (SRC) sine scleroderma. Fortunately this is a rare condition but renal crisis can precede the onset of skin disease. The presence of nail bed capillary loop abnormalities, high-titer ANA, new onset renal failure, malignant hypertension, and microangiopathic hemolysis is classic for this condition. High-dose corticosteroids are associated with SRC and should be avoided in patients with known scleroderma. Aggressive early use of angiotensin converting inhibitors (ACE) is warranted for renal protection.

Steen VD. Scleroderma renal crisis. Rheum Dis Clin North Am. 1996;22:861–78.

Steen VD, Medsger TA Jr. Case-control study of corticosteroids and other drugs that either precipitate or protect from the development of scleroderma renal crisis. Arthritis Rheum. 1998;41: 1613–19.

Question 14

A 19-year-old previously healthy student is evaluated for new onset fever, joint pain, and rash. She is sexually active but denies diarrhea, urethral discharge, or sore throat. Her symptoms occurred 1 week following her menses. There was no history of travel, tick bite, or prior joint symptoms. Physical examination reveals a febrile patient with pustular lesions over the arms and tenosynovitis of the wrist. Her immunologic and hematologic studies and renal parameters are normal. The laboratory calls to inform you of gram negative diplococci growing in the blood cultures.

What is the diagnosis and how would you treat her?

Yousaf Ali, *Self Assessment Questions in Rheumatology,* DOI: 10.1007/ 978-1-59745-497-1,
Humana Press, a part of Springer Science+Business Media, LLC 2009

Answer: Disseminated gonococcal arthritis (DGI)

This patient has the classic arthritis–dermatitis syndrome characterized by teno-synovitis and purulent vesicles. DGI is more common in women, and menstruation appears to be an important risk factor. The diagnosis is established by culturing the blood, cervix, urethra, rectum, pharynx, and synovial fluid. The patient and her partner should also receive testing for chlamydia.

Treatment for DGI is an intravenous cephalosporin regimen (e.g., ceftriaxone 1 g IV every 8 h) until clinical improvement followed by an oral cephalosporin.

CDC. Updated regimens, April 2007 – STD Treatment Guidelines 2006. **CDC, Atlanta, GA.**

Rice PA. Gonococcal arthritis (disseminated gonococcal infection). Infect Dis Clin North Am. 2005 Dec;19(4):853-61. Review.

Question 15

A 77-year-old male is referred to you for the treatment of intercritical gout. His serum UA is 12.5 mg/dl and he has mild renal insufficiency with a serum creatinine of 1.6 mg/dl. Allopurinol and once daily colchicine are prescribed.

He calls your answering service 1 week later with new onset of fatigue and ecchymosis.

What complication has occurred?

Yousaf Ali, *Self Assessment Questions in Rheumatology,* DOI: 10.1007/ 978-1-59745-497-1,
Humana Press, a part of Springer Science + Business Media, LLC 2009

Answer: This patient has most likely developed allopurinol-associated aplastic anemia

This condition occurs rarely and may be more common in patients with renal failure. Allopurinol should be immediately discontinued and hematologic support instituted. Although colchicine toxicity can also cause bone marrow failure this tends to occur with higher doses.

Conrad ME. Fatal aplastic anemia associated with allopurinol therapy. Am J Hematol. 1986 May;22(1):107–8.

Lin YW, Okazaki S, Hamahata K, Watanabe K, Usami I, Yoshibayashi M, Akiyama Y, Kubota M. Acute pure red cell aplasia associated with allopurinol therapy. Am J Hematol. 1999 Jul;61(3):209–11.

Shinohara K, Okafuji K, Ayame H, Tanaka M. Aplastic anemia caused by allopurinol in renal insufficiency. Am J Hematol. 1990 Sep;35(1):68.

Question 16

A 35-year-old female is seen for follow-up of Sjogrens syndrome due to persistent arthritis and parotitis. You consider starting azathioprine. She informs you that her sister took this medicine and had a "bad reaction with her blood."

What tests should be ordered prior to commencing this drug?
How common is this abnormality?

Yousaf Ali, *Self Assessment Questions in Rheumatology,* DOI: 10.1007/ 978-1-59745-497-1,
Humana Press, a part of Springer Science+Business Media, LLC 2009

Answer: Thiopurine *S*-methyltransferase (TPMT) mutation

This is inherited as an autosomal dominant trait. The estimated prevalence of TPMT intermediate activity is about 10% although 1 in 300 people are homozygous for the gene mutation. Since TPMT activity is required to metabolize thiopurine drugs a deficiency can result in severe myelosuppression.

Krynetski EY, Evans WE. Genetic polymorphism of thiopurine *S*-methyltransferase: molecular mechanisms and clinical importance. Pharmacology 2000;61:136–46.

Question 17

A 31-year-old African American male is seen for evaluation of uveitis and bell's palsy. He has a low-grade fever, parotid gland enlargement, mild arthritis, and dyspnea on exertion.

What is the most likely diagnosis?
What treatment is indicated?

Yousaf Ali, *Self Assessment Questions in Rheumatology,* DOI: 10.1007/ 978-1-59745-497-1,
Humana Press, a part of Springer Science + Business Media, LLC 2009

Answer: Heerfordt's syndrome

This patient has sarcoidosis with involvement of the uveal tract and parotid gland. Ninety percent of patients with sarcoidosis have pulmonary involvement, and further evaluation should include chest radiography with pulmonary function testing. The goal of treatment is to decrease inflammation and the mainstay of treatment is corticosteroids. Ocular inflammation often responds to topical steroids. Sarcoidosis is often a self-limiting disease.

White ES, Lynch JP III. Current and emerging strategies for the management of sarcoidosis. Expert Opin Pharmacother. 2007 Jun;8(9):1293–311. Review.

Question 18

A 76-year-old male is referred for further management of ankylosing spondylitis. He was told he had a "bamboo spine" on routine CXR. He emphatically denies stiffness, pain, or enthesopathy. His examination shows slightly limited spine flexion, normal chest excursion, and wall-to-occiput distance of 2 in. Inflammatory markers are not elevated and he had no history of ocular disease or adolescent back pain.

What is the most likely diagnosis?
What other tests will facilitate the diagnosis?
What treatment is advised?

Yousaf Ali, *Self Assessment Questions in Rheumatology,* DOI: 10.1007/ 978-1-59745-497-1,
Humana Press, a part of Springer Science+Business Media, LLC 2009

Answer:

1. Diffuse idiopathic hyperostosis syndrome (DISH). It is very unlikely that the patient has ankylosing spondylitis (AS). AS typically affects young men in the second and third decade of life and is characterized by stiffness of the axial skeleton and sacroiliac joints. This elderly gentleman most likely has DISH syndrome, which is a condition that involves flowing ossifications along the anterolateral aspect of four contiguous vertebra. It is of unknown etiology but usually involves the thoracic spine.

2. HLA-B27 gene is present in 95% of patients with AS. A pelvic radiograph would demonstrate the absence of sacroiliac disease in DISH syndrome.

3. No treatment is indicated.

Atzeni F, Sarzi-Puttini P, Bevilacqua M. Calcium deposition and associated chronic diseases (atherosclerosis, diffuse idiopathic skeletal hyperostosis, and others). Rheum Dis Clin North Am. 2006 May;32(2):413–26, viii. Review.

Question 19

A 73-year-old male is referred for evaluation of refractory lower extremity edema. He has had slight stiffness in the proximal areas but is more concerned about his leg swelling. He denies headaches/jaw claudication or visual changes. On examination he has small joint synovitis and 3+ pitting peripheral edema. There are no signs of heart failure.

Investigations reveal normal renal function and urinalysis. Hb = 11.1 g/dl, ESR = 45 mm/h. RF/CCP antibody are negative. Ultrasound of the LE reveals no evidence of venous occlusion. A two-dimensional ECHO is normal without pericardial or right-sided dysfunction.

What is the most likely diagnosis?
What treatment is advised?
What is the prognosis?

Yousaf Ali, *Self Assessment Questions in Rheumatology,* DOI: 10.1007/ 978-1-59745-497-1,
Humana Press, a part of Springer Science + Business Media, LLC 2009

Answer: Remitting seronegative symmetrical synovitis with peripheral edema (RS3PE)

This patient has classic RS3PE with peripheral edema and symmetrical swelling but no evidence of RA. This is a rare condition that mimicks PMR and RA although there are no long-term consequences of joint damage or deformity. Patients often have modestly elevated inflammatory markers and respond well to oral corticosteroids. Prognosis is generally excellent.

Olivieri I, Salvarani C, Cantini F. RS3PE syndrome: an overview.
Clin Exp Rheumatol. 2000 Jul/Aug;18(4 Suppl 20):S53–S55. Review.

Question 20

A 47-year-old female presents with arthralgia, rash, and parasthesias. Her examination reveals palpable purpura and peripheral neuropathy but no synovitis. She denies xerostomia, sicca symptoms, renal disease, or recurrent sinusitis. Her laboratory tests reveal modest transaminitis with low serum albumin, prolonged prothrombin time. ANA is negative but RF is moderately positive. ANCA tests are negative.

What is the most likely diagnosis?

Yousaf Ali, *Self Assessment Questions in Rheumatology,* DOI: 10.1007/ 978-1-59745-497-1, Humana Press, a part of Springer Science + Business Media, LLC 2009

Answer: Hepatitis C virus (HCV) with mixed cryoglobulinemia

This patient has evidence of chronic liver disease with decreased synthetic function. The constellation of palpable purpura, arthralgia, and neuropathy are highly suggestive of mixed croglubulinemia (MC). MC is quite common in HCV although only clinically apparent in about 10% of patients. It is also associated with membranoproliferative glomerulonephritis and vasculitis.

Saadoun D, Landau DA, Calabrese LH, Cacoub PP. Hepatitis C-associated mixed cryoglobulinaemia: a crossroad between autoimmunity and lymphoproliferation. Rheumatology. 2007 Aug; 46(8):1234–42.

Question 21

A 21-year-old patient returns from New England following a trip and is referred for arthralgia, flu-like symptoms, headache, and malaise. His examination is nonfocal apart from a fever of 100.2°F. Laboratory data reveal Hb = 12.3 g/dl, WBC = 2.8, and platelets = 25K. Wright Giemsa staining of the peripheral smear reveals morula within the neutrophils. Biochemical parameters are normal apart from a slight elevation of the LDH.

What is the most likely diagnosis?
How would you treat this?
What other conditions need to be considered?

Yousaf Ali, *Self Assessment Questions in Rheumatology*, DOI: 10.1007/ 978-1-59745-497-1,
Humana Press, a part of Springer Science+Business Media, LLC 2009

Answer: Human granulocytic anaplasmosis (formerly ehrlichiosis) (HGA)

HGA is becoming a more commonly recognized cause of fever following a tick bite in the USA. The vector for this infection is the Ixodes tick, which also carries the spirochaete responsible for lyme disease (*Borrelia Burgdorferi*). Humans are affected when they impinge on small mammal/tick-infested areas. The common clinical presentation is fever, headache, and myalgia. Arthralgias, septic shock, pancytopenia, renal failure, and acute respiratory distress syndrome (ARDS) are also rare complications. Treatment is with oral doxycycline.

Coinfection with babesiosis and lyme disease can also occur and should be checked in symptomatic patients who live in endemic areas.

Wormser GP, Dattwyler RJ, Shapiro ED, Halperin JJ, Steere AC, Klempner MS, Krause PJ, Bakken JS, Strle F, Stanek G, Bockenstedt L, Fish D, Dumler JS, Nadelman RB. Infectious Diseases Society of America practice guidelines for clinical assessment, treatment and prevention of lyme disease, human granulocytic anaplasmosis, and babesiosis. Clin Infect Dis. 2006 Nov 1;43(9):1089–1134.

Question 22

A 44-year-old well-nourished Caucasian female is referred for evaluation of a swollen knee. She has presented to the ER on two occasions and had the knee drained. Serial culture results are negative and no crystals have been observed. The effusions have been "bloody" although she denies trauma or anticoagulant use. She walks with a limp and is otherwise well without systemic complaints. On examination she has a swollen right knee with boggy synovial thickening and mild warmth. No other joints are involved. A knee radiograph is normal. Lab tests including ANA, RF, ESR, and lyme serology are negative. Hematologic studies are normal.

What is the most likely diagnosis?
How would you manage this patient?
What relevance is her state of nourishment?

Yousaf Ali, *Self Assessment Questions in Rheumatology,* DOI: 10.1007/ 978-1-59745-497-1,
Humana Press, a part of Springer Science+Business Media, LLC 2009

Answer: Pigmented villonodular synovitis (PVNS)

The differential diagnosis for a hemarthrosis includes bleeding diathesis, trauma, pseudogout, charcot joint, and PVNS. Since her hematologic indices are normal and there has been no trauma; intraarticular hemorrhage or charcot joint seem less likely. Pseudogout is typically seen in older patients with preexisting degenerative joint disease, metabolic disease, or hyperparathyroidism, and no crystals have been observed.

PVNS is a rare slow-growing benign tumor of the synovium with typical MRI findings. Treatment is arthroscopic synovectomy.

Her nourishment is relevant as scurvy can also cause recurrent hemarthrosis.

Fain O. Musculoskeletal manifestations of scurvy. Joint Bone Spine. 2005 Mar;72(2):124–8.

Mendenhall WM, Mendenhall CM, Reith JD, Scarborough MT, Gibbs CP, Mendenhall NP. Pigmented villonodular synovitis. Am J Clin Oncol. 2006 Dec;29(6):548–50. Review.

Question 23

A 78-year-old female is referred for treatment of osteoporosis. She has a history of breast cancer in situ without skeletal involvement, and esophageal reflux. Axial T scores are −2.6, Hip −2.7.

On examination she has bilateral poor dentition and marked kyphoscoliosis. There is a history of hip and spine fracture. Calcium, vitamin D, PTH, and renal function are normal. Her breast cancer is currently in remission.

Her GP has tried both residronate and alendronate, which caused GI distress.

How would you manage her osteoporosis.
What drugs should be avoided?

Yousaf Ali, *Self Assessment Questions in Rheumatology,* DOI: 10.1007/ 978-1-59745-497-1,
Humana Press, a part of Springer Science + Business Media, LLC 2009

Answer: Subcutaneous teriperatide would be a good choice as it is an anabolic agent that avoids the oral route

This patient is at a moderately high risk for future fracture. The most potent oral antiresorptive agents are bisphosphonates (BP), which have been shown to decrease incident vertebral and hip fractures. Unfortunately, because of her esophageal disease she is a poor candidate for BPs, which can cause GI distress. A selective estrogen modulator (SERM) such as raloxifene would be a reasonable choice given her prior breast cancer although there are no data to support a reduction in hip fracture.

Teriperatide is an anabolic agent used in patients refractory to oral agents at high risk for fracture. It is given via the subcutaneous route and generally well tolerated in patients with esophageal issues.

Intravenous bisphosphonates should be avoided in this patient given the higher incidence of osteonecrosis of the jaw (ONJ) in patients with preexisting poor dentition, malignancy, diabetes, and nicotine use.

Bamias A, Kastritis E, Bamia C, et al. Osteonecrosis of the jaw in cancer treatment after bisphosphonates: incidence and risk factors. J Clin Oncol. 2005;34:8580–7.

Durie BGM, Katz M, Crowley J. Osteonecrosis of the jaw and bisphosphonates. N Engl J Med. 2005;353:99–102.

Question 24

A 46-year-old diabetic male has pain over the metacarpophalangeal (MCP) joints. He has about 15 min of morning stiffness. On examination he has swollen tender second/third mcp joints but no overt synovitis.

Serologies are negative and radiographs reveal hook-like osteophytes at the MCP and PIP joints.

What is the most likely diagnosis?
What tests would you order?

Yousaf Ali, *Self Assessment Questions in Rheumatology,* DOI: 10.1007/ 978-1-59745-497-1,
Humana Press, a part of Springer Science + Business Media, LLC 2009

Answer: Hemochromatosis

An elevated ferritin or transferrin saturation is suggestive of hemochromatosis. Patients develop osteoarthritis of the second and third MCP joint, which may be the initial clue to the diagnosis. Iron deposition occurs in the pancreas causing diabetes. Occasionally, chondrocalcinosis is observed.

Jordan JM. Arthritis in hemochromatosis or iron storage disease. Curr Opin Rheumatol. 2004 Jan;16(1):62–6. Review.

Question 25

A 46-year-old smoker is referred with painful shins. She has a normal examination apart from a right-sided horner's syndrome. Radiographs of the tibia and fibula are normal

What is the next appropriate test to confirm the diagnosis?

Yousaf Ali, *Self Assessment Questions in Rheumatology*, DOI: 10.1007/ 978-1-59745-497-1,
Humana Press, a part of Springer Science + Business Media, LLC 2009

Answer: Chest X-ray

This patient most likely has a Pancoast's tumor causing hypertrophic pulmonary oste-oarthropathy (HPOA). Bronchogenic carcinoma is one of the causes of HPOA and results in periostitis and clubbing. Although the cause is unknown, abnormal expression of vascular endothelial growth factor (VEGF) has been described in this condition.

Martinez-Lavin M. Exploring the cause of the most ancient clinical sign of medicine: finger clubbing. Semin Arthritis Rheum. 2007 Jun;36(6):380–5.

Question 26

A 78-year-old female is seen due to a swollen right shoulder. She denies having trauma or prior history of crystal arthritis. Her shoulder examination reveals a large warm effusion with limitation of motion in all directions. A radiograph demonstrates advanced glenohumeral destruction but no calcification. Arthrocentesis reveals a bloody effusion without evidence of infection or crystals on conventional polarized microscopy; cytology is negative.

What test should you order from your laboratory that will most likely yield the diagnosis?

Yousaf Ali, *Self Assessment Questions in Rheumatology*, DOI: 10.1007/ 978-1-59745-497-1, Humana Press, a part of Springer Science + Business Media, LLC 2009

Answer: Alizarin Stain

This patient most likely has Milwaukee shoulder due to the presence of calcium hydroxyapatite crystals. This condition is characterized by intrarticular or peri-articular hydroxyapatite crystals causing a destructive arthropathy at the gleno-humeral and rotator cuff interval. The cause is unknown.

Ea HK, Lioté F. Calcium pyrophosphate dihydrate and basic calcium phosphate crystal-induced arthropathies: update on pathogenesis, clinical features, and therapy. Curr Rheumatol Rep. 2004 Jun;6(3):221–7. Review.

Question 27

A 19-year-old female with SLE presents with a new limp and right groin pain. One week prior to presentation she received high-dose intravenous corticosteroids for class IV glomerulonephritis.

On examination there are no findings apart from irritation of the right hip with rotation. A pelvic and hip radiograph are normal.

What is the most likely diagnosis? How would you manage the patient?

Yousaf Ali, *Self Assessment Questions in Rheumatology*, DOI: 10.1007/ 978-1-59745-497-1,
Humana Press, a part of Springer Science+Business Media, LLC 2009

Answer: Avascular necrosis (AVN) of the femoral head

AVN results in dead trabecular bone and marrow extending to involve the subchondral plate due to local ischemia. The highest incidence of AVN of the hips occurs in patients with SLE and renal transplants, who have been exposed to high-dose steroids. Ultimately collapse of the femoral head occurs, which necessitates hip replacement. In early stage 1 AVN plain radiographs are normal and so a high level of suspicion needs to be maintained.

The patient should be evaluated by an orthopedist and avoid weight-bearing. Core decompression should be considered depending on the severity of necrosis. Since the risk of AVN is greater in patients with hypercoagulability, antiphospholipid syndrome should be excluded.

Abu-Shakra M, Buskila D, Shoenfeld Y. Osteonecrosis in patients with SLE. Clin Rev Allergy Immunol. 2003 Aug;25(1):13–24. Review.

Question 28

A 65-year-old female is referred by the GP due to an elevated creatinine phosphokinase (CPK). She has a history of obstructive sleep apnea, type 2 diabetes, and hypertension. There is no history of trauma, intramuscular injection, or dark urine. Recently she was started on atorvastatin 20 mg daily. A routine blood test 1 month after the lab test revealed a CPK of 525 IU/ml (nl < 250); no baseline level is available. On examination, she is obese; weight 350 lb. There are no rashes, nodules, or muscle tenderness. Muscle strength is 5/5 throughout

What additional blood tests would you like to know?
What management is indicated?

Yousaf Ali, *Self Assessment Questions in Rheumatology,* DOI: 10.1007/ 978-1-59745-497-1,
Humana Press, a part of Springer Science + Business Media, LLC 2009

Answer: TSH, renal function

This patient has a slightly elevated CPK level without symptoms of muscle break-down or inflammation. Given her obesity, the most likely scenario is that the CPK reflects her high muscle mass and is normal when calibrated for her BMI.

This is a common scenario in practice and in the absence of weakness, rhab-domyolysis, or pain no specific treatment is indicated. Given her cardiac risk fac-tors she should continue the statin therapy and the CPK levels should be monitored closely.

A TSH should be checked to exclude hypothyroid myopathy. Renal function should also be checked as rhabdomyolysis is a serious complication of muscle breakdown and needs to be excluded. The absence of arthritis, Raynaud's pheno-menon, or rash makes a connective tissue less likely.

Question 29

A 28-year-old female patient is referred for osteoporosis. She has a 6-month history of weakness, myalgia, and 50-lb weight gain. Three months prior, she fell and fractured her pelvis. PMH is unremarkable apart from poorly controlled hypertension. Her menses are normal. She takes no medications apart from atenolol.

Lab work reveals K = 3.2 meq, normal renal and hematologic parameters. CPK, vitamin D, and malabsorption studies including celiac antibodies are normal. A bone DEXA scan reveals an axial T score of −3.5 and hip T score of −3.3. Corresponding Z scores are both less than −2.0.

Her examination reveals a bitemporal hemianopsia, BP 155/95, obesity, and mild muscle tenderness.

What is the most likely diagnosis?
What is the optimal treatment?

Yousaf Ali, *Self Assessment Questions in Rheumatology,* DOI: 10.1007/ 978-1-59745-497-1,
Humana Press, a part of Springer Science + Business Media, LLC 2009

Answer: Cushing's disease secondary to pituitary adenoma with suprasellar extension

Excessive cortisol production from an ACTH-secreting tumor results in hypertension, hypokalemia, and accelerated osteoporosis. A large mass that extends into the suprasellar fossa can place pressure on the optic chiasma resulting in visual field defects. In this case prolonged exposure of cortisol has resulted in osteoporosis. A low Z score below −2.0 raises the possibility of age inappropriate low bone mass.

The treatment of choice for classic Cushing's disease is surgical resection of the adenoma with the goal being to relieve pressure and preserve pituitary function.

Newell-Price J, Bertagna X, Grossman AB, Nieman LK. Cushing's syndrome. Lancet. 2006 May 13;367(9522):1605–17. Review.

Question 30

A 32-year-old teacher presents with refractory left-sided Raynaud's and left-sided neck pain. She has no other serologic or clinical stigmata of a connective tissue disease. Treatment with calcium channel blockers, aspirin, nitrates, and alpha blockers is ineffective. Her examination reveals a diminished left radial pulse with inspiration.
Blood work is normal.

What is the most likely diagnosis?

Yousaf Ali, *Self Assessment Questions in Rheumatology,* DOI: 10.1007/ 978-1-59745-497-1,
Humana Press, a part of Springer Science+Business Media, LLC 2009

Answer: Thoracic outlet syndrome due to cervical rib

This young patient has unilateral evidence of vascular insufficiency in the upper extremity. In a nonsmoker the differential diagnosis includes Raynaud's phenomenon or occlusion of the subclavian artery. Usual causes of Raynaud's phenomenon include idiopathic, hyperviscosity, atherosclerosis, connective tissue disease, or vasculitis. These are less likely in this case since the symptoms are unilateral. The patient has a positive Adson's maneuver with a diminishing pulse on inspiration suggestive of a cervical rib or fibrous band.

A CXR with apical lordotic view will show the cervical rib.

Mackinnon SE, Novak CB. Thoracic outlet syndrome. Curr Probl Surg. 2002 Nov;39(11):1070–145. Review.

Question 31

You are asked to see a 22-year-old female from Laos who is admitted as an inpatient. She presented with a febrile illness with quotidian spikes to 101°F. There is associated malaise and general weakness. There has been no recent travel out of the USA for over a year and no sick contacts, tick bites, or rash. On examination she is febrile, and there is diffuse shotty lymphadenopathy, splenomegaly, and bilateral warm knee effusions. Her lab work reveals leukocytosis with lymphocytic predominance, normal renal function, mild transaminitis, and low serum albumin. Urinalysis is normal with no proteinuria or cellular activity. Microbiologic, viral, and rickettsial titers are negative. Bone marrow studies are nondiagnostic and negative for mycobacteria. CT scans of abdomen, chest, and pelvis are normal.

You order blood work: ANA +1:40, RF negative, CCP negative, ASO, Parvovirus, and urine tests for gonorrhea are negative. ESR is 115 mm, CRP = 372 mg/dl, and ferritin = 4,500 ng/ml.

What is the most likely diagnosis?
How would you manage her?

Yousaf Ali, *Self Assessment Questions in Rheumatology,* DOI: 10.1007/ 978-1-59745-497-1,
Humana Press, a part of Springer Science+Business Media, LLC 2009

Answer: The most likely diagnosis is adult onset Still's disease (AOSD)

This patient has the classic features of AOSD with spiking fever, organomegaly, derangement of liver function, leukocytosis, and a very high ferritin. This is a tricky diagnosis due to the broad differential diagnosis and potential range of infections or malignancies that can present with this type of presentation. One of the more specific clues lies in the serum ferritin, which is usually markedly elevated in AOSD and often >3,000 ng/ml. The differential diagnosis of a very high ferritin (>1,000 ng/ml) is limited to hemochromatosis, hemophagocytic syndrome, or AOSD.

Once infection and malignancy have been excluded treatment with high-dose steroids should be initiated in this patient who is sick with this multisystem disease. For mild flares nonsteroidal drugs may be used.

Efthimiou P, Georgy S. Pathogenesis and management of adult-onset Still's disease. Semin Arthritis Rheum. 2006 Dec;36(3):144–152.

Zandman-Goddard G, Shoenfeld Y. Ferritin in autoimmune diseases. Autoimmun Rev. 2007 Aug;6(7):457–63.

Question 32

A 75-year-old man is referred to evaluate an elevated ESR. He has had occipital and bitemporal HA of 3-months duration with associated jaw pain and scalp tenderness. A 1-cm left temporal biopsy is negative for temporal arteritis or vasculitis. On examination he appears cachectic and has diffuse tenderness over the right temporal artery. There is lymphadenopathy and right-sided diplopia with medial rectus weakness.

Labs reveal normocytic anemia, ESR = 88mm/hr. Hepatic and renal functions are intact. Immunoelectrophoresis is without monoclonality.

What tests would you order to confirm the diagnosis?

Yousaf Ali, *Self Assessment Questions in Rheumatology*, DOI: 10.1007/ 978-1-59745-497-1,
Humana Press, a part of Springer Science + Business Media, LLC 2009

Answer: Bilateral 4–6 cm TA biopsy

This elderly gentleman has symptoms that are classic for temporal arteritis (TA). Headaches and jaw claudication in the setting of a markedly elevated ESR should raise suspicion for TA. Unfortunately this is a disease of discontinuity and characterized by skip lesions on TA biopsy. Ideally a 4–6-cm biopsy should be obtained and a bilateral biopsy will increase the sensitivity, albeit marginally. In this case the 1-cm biopsy length is inadequate.

TA responds to high-dose prednisone and untreated can cause optic arteritis resulting in blindness. Opthalmoplegia has also been described. Myasthenia gravis or a space-occupying lesion would not cause bilateral headaches, jaw claudication, or scalp tenderness. If the clinical suspicion is high and an inadequate biopsy is obtained it should be repeated. Another option would be to obtain a color duplex ultrasound, which, in the right hands, can reveal a "halo" sign that is suggestive of active arteritis.

Butteriss DJ, Clarke L, Dayan M, Birchall D. Use of colour duplex ultrasound to diagnose giant cell arteritis in a case of visual loss of uncertain aetiology. Br J Radiol. 2004 Jul;77(919):607–9.

Lazaridis C, Torabi A, Cannon S. Bilateral third nerve palsy and temporal arteritis. Arch Neurol. 2005 Nov;62(11):1766–8. Review.

Pless M, Rizzo JF III, Lamkin JC, Lessell S. Concordance of bilateral temporal artery biopsy in giant cell arteritis. J Neuroophthalmol. 2000 Sep;20(3):216–18.

Salvarani C, Cantini F, Boiardi L, Hunder GG. Polymyalgia rheumatica and giant-cell arteritis. N Engl J Med. 2002 Jul 25;347(4):261–71. Review.

Seo P, Stone JH. Large-vessel vasculitis. Arthritis Rheum. 2004 Feb 15;51(1):128–39. Review.

Question 33

A 46-year-old male is admitted with new onset of rectal bleeding after having taken 1,600-mg ibuprofen for an acutely swollen toe. You are asked to examine him by the colorectal surgeon for acute podagra. They are considering a colectomy to arrest the bleeding, which has failed to stop by conventional means.

On examination he has a red tender inflamed first toe with exquisite tenderness. Lab work reveals mild anemia, mild prerenal kidney dysfunction. Uric acid is normal.

How would you treat his gout?

Yousaf Ali, *Self Assessment Questions in Rheumatology*, DOI: 10.1007/ 978-1-59745-497-1,
Humana Press, a part of Springer Science + Business Media, LLC 2009

Answer: Intraarticular (IA) corticosteroid injection

This patient has acute podagra in the setting of an acute NSAID-induced gastrointestinal bleed. An IA injection of steroid is the optimal management in this patient. Colchicine is contraindicated given the renal impairment and potential to further irritate the GI tract.

Keith MP, Gilliland WR. Updates in the management of gout.
Am J Med. 2007 Mar;120(3):221–4. Review.

Question 34

A 22-year-old male presents with recurrent intermittent monoarthritis affecting the toes, knees, and ankle. Arthrocentesis reveals intracellular uric acid crystals diagnostic of acute gout. Lab work: Cr = 0.6 mg/dl, UA = 14 mg/dl, CBC normal. Hepatic function is normal. Twenty-four hour urine UA is low.

What is the most likely diagnosis and cause?

Yousaf Ali, *Self Assessment Questions in Rheumatology*, DOI: 10.1007/ 978-1-59745-497-1, Humana Press, a part of Springer Science + Business Media, LLC 2009

Answer: Congenital under excretion of uric acid (UA) due to a tubular defect

The majority of people with gout are congenital underexcretors of UA. The exact mechanism has not been elucidated but it is related to decreased secretion, increased reabsorption, or decreased filtration of UA. Overproduction of UA occurs in less than 10% of patients. Lesch Nyhan syndrome secondary to hypoxanthine guanine phosphoribosyl transferase deficiency (HGPRT) would cause an overproduction of UA and increased 24-h urinary uric acid excretion.

Emmerson BT, Nagel SL, Duffy DL, Martin NG. Genetic control of the renal clearance of urate: a study of twins. Ann Rheum Dis. 1992;51:375.

Lesch M, Nyhan WL. A familial disorder of uric acid metabolism and central nervous system function. Am J Med. 1964;36:561.

Question 35

A 45-year-old female with 10 years of seropositive erosive rheumatoid arthritis presents with new onset of shortness of breath, low-grade fever, and dry cough. Her current regimen includes hydroxychloroquine 400 mg/day, prednisone 10 mg/day, sulfasalazine 3 g daily, and infliximab 5 mg/kg. She has never taken methotrexate. She resides in New England, and denies recent travel.

Examination reveals chronic rheumatoid deformities without active synovitis. Pulmonary examination reveals fine diffuse inspiratory crepitations bilaterally. A CXR describes fine perihilar reticular opacification. Blood gases revealed hypoxia, and she failed to improve with broad spectrum and empiric macrolide therapy. Lab work reveals normocytic anemia without leucocytosis. Renal, liver function and CPK are normal. LDH is markedly elevated. Peripheral smear is without hemolysis.

Bronchoscopy reveals negative stains for acid- and alcohol-fast bacilli on three occasions and PPD (TB) skin tests are negative. CMV, *Mycoplasma*, *Legionella*, Q-fever, adenovirus, influenza, *Chlamydia*, cytomegalovirus, Epstein-Barr virus, hepatitis B and C, and HIV titers are negative.

What is the most likely diagnosis?

Yousaf Ali, *Self Assessment Questions in Rheumatology*, DOI: 10.1007/ 978-1-59745-497-1,
Humana Press, a part of Springer Science + Business Media, LLC 2009

Answer: Pneumocystis jiroveci (carinii) pneumonia (PCP)

This patient who is receiving anti-TNF therapy presents with an acute pulmonary decompensation characterized by dyspnea, hypoxemia, and an elevated LDH level. Since she is significantly immunosuppressed, an opportunistic infection is the most likely scenario. Rheumatoid lung disease, bronchiolitis obliterans with organizing pneumonia (BOOP) are also in the differential diagnosis. RA-associated lung disease tends to present more insidiously with pleural involvement and is usually not associated with elevated LDH levels.

PCP is caused by a unicellular eukaryote and is a rare cause of infection in immunocompetent individuals. The diagnostic gold standard is a broncheoalveolar lavage (BAL) with cytologic confirmation of induced sputum samples. LDH levels are a sensitive but poorly specific indicator of PCP. Since this infection is associated with high mortality a high index of suspicion is required.

Butt AA, Michaels S, Kissinger P. The association of serum lactate dehydrogenase level with selected opportunistic infections and HIV progression. Int J Infect Dis. 2002 Sep;6(3):178–81.

Kaur N, Mahl TC. Pneumocystis jiroveci (carinii) pneumonia after infliximab therapy: a review of 84 cases. Dig Dis Sci. 2007 Jun;52(6):1481–4.

Mutlu GM, Mutlu EA, Bellmeyer A, Rubinstein I. Pulmonary adverse events of anti-tumor necrosis factor-alpha antibody therapy. Am J Med. 2006 Aug;119(8):639–46. Review.

Question 36

A 44-year-old female presents with recurrent uveitis and scleritis. She has a 3-month history of nasal discharge and shortness of breath. CXR is reported as having cavitatory lesions. Nasal mucosa is erythematous and reveals a perforation within the septum. She has no evidence of synovitis, rash, or mononeuritis on examination. Microbiologic evaluation, including TB and cocaine use is negative. PFTs reveal mild restriction and upper airway obstruction.

What is the most likely diagnosis and how would you make this diagnosis?

Yousaf Ali, *Self Assessment Questions in Rheumatology,* DOI: 10.1007/ 978-1-59745-497-1,
Humana Press, a part of Springer Science + Business Media, LLC 2009

Answer: Wegener's granulomatosis (WG)

This patient presents with recurrent sinusitis, inflammatory eye disease, and cavitatory lung lesions typical for WG. The definitive diagnosis is made by confirming the presence of noncaseating granulomas on biopsy. Serological tests include the presence of antineutrophil cytoplasmic antibodies (c-ANCA), which have a sensitivity of about 60–88%. Antibodies to proteinase 3 (PR-3) are highly sensitive in active WG (90%). Other features of WG include subglottic stenosis, pauciimmune glomerulonephritis, mononeuritis multiplex, and arthritis. In this patient other causes of cavitatory lung lesions such as infection need to be excluded prior to treatment.

Bosch X, Guilabert A, Font J. Antineutrophil cytoplasmic antibodies. Lancet. 2006 Jul 29;368(9533):404–18. Review.

Seo P, Stone JH. The antineutrophil cytoplasmic antibody-associated vasculitides. Am J Med. 2004 Jul 1;117(1):39–50. Review.

Question 37

A 33-year-old heterosexual monogamous firefighter is referred for bloody diarrhea and new onset of knee swelling. He is stiff for about 45 min in the morning. There is no history of travel, urethral discharge, or uveitis. On examination he has a warm left knee effusion and mild tenderness in the abdomen. Spine forward flexion is slightly limited. A painful erythematous rash is noted on the anterior shins. Lab work reveals mild microcytic anemia. ESR is 110 mm/h. Stool cultures are negative. Renal and hepatic function is preserved.

What is the most likely diagnosis and how would you confirm it? How would you initially manage his joint pain?

Yousaf Ali, *Self Assessment Questions in Rheumatology,* DOI: 10.1007/ 978-1-59745-497-1,
Humana Press, a part of Springer Science+Business Media, LLC 2009

Answer: Inflammatory bowel disease-related arthropathy

This gentleman presents with a syndrome of bloody diarrhea, erythema nodosum, and oligoarthritis. This pattern is most classic for inflammatory bowel disease (IBD). Ideally his knee should be drained and fluid sent to confirm a sterile effusion. Colonoscopy with biopsy will confirm the diagnosis of IBD.

Initial treatment of his joint disease can involve local intraarticular injections, analgesic medications, and judicious use of anti-inflammatory medications with close collaboration with the gastroenterologist. Axial spondylitis may respond to physical therapy. The response to DMARD therapy for peripheral and axial arthritis is often disappointing. Monoclonal antibody anti-TNF agents (infliximab and adalimumab), in contrast, work well in this situation.

Padovan M, Castellino G, Govoni M, Trotta F. The treatment of the rheumatological manifestations of the inflammatory bowel diseases. Rheumatol Int. 2006 Sep;26(11):953–8. Review.

Van den Bosch F, Kruithof E, De Vos M, De Keyser F, Mielants H. Crohn's disease associated with spondyloarthropathy: effect of TNF-alpha blockade with infliximab on articular symptoms. Lancet. 2000 Nov 25;356(9244):1821–2.

Question 38

A 67-year-old female with RA is referred for further management. She has multiple comorbidities including chronic renal failure, diabetes, and hypertension. She has pain in the hands, wrists, and feet with 4 h of early morning stiffness. On examination there is polyarthritis of the small joints of the hands with significant joint margin tenderness. Prednisone at 15 mg daily and weekly methotrexate (MTX) at 15 mg is commenced. You are called by the ER 1 week later where she is being seen for new onset odonophagia and dysphagia. On examination she has severe mucosal ulceration. Lab work reveals mild hyperglycemia and stable renal dysfunction.

What complication has occurred?
How could this have been prevented?

Yousaf Ali, *Self Assessment Questions in Rheumatology*, DOI: 10.1007/ 978-1-59745-497-1,
Humana Press, a part of Springer Science + Business Media, LLC 2009

Answer: MTX mucositis

This patient with renal failure has developed mucositis from the methotrexate. Mucosal toxicity is a well-known complication of MTX and predisposing factors include folate deficiency, renal failure, and hypoalbuminemia. There are also various genetic polymorphisms that may predict toxicity and response to MTX. The dose of MTX should be adjusted in patients with renal failure.

This complication may have been prevented by the use of a lower dose and prophylactic daily folic acid.

Grosflam J, Weinblatt ME. Methotrexate: mechanism of action, pharmacokinetics, clinical indications, and toxicity. Curr Opin Rheumatol. 1991 Jun;3(3):363–8. Review.

Takatori R, Takahashi KA, Tokunaga D, Hojo T, Fujioka M, Asano T, Hirata T, Kawahito Y, Satomi Y, Nishino H, Tanaka T, Hirota Y, Kubo T. ABCB1 C3435T polymorphism influences methotrexate sensitivity in rheumatoid arthritis patients. Clin Exp Rheumatol. 2006 Sep/Oct;24(5):546–54.

Question 39

A 68-year-old Caucasian female is referred for further management of osteoporosis. She underwent early menopause at 43 and did not receive hormone replacement. A bone density taken 2 years before revealed an axial T score of 0.5 and appendicular T score of −2.6. She was treated with calcium supplements and alendronate 70 mg weekly. Despite bisphosphonate therapy she has had several fragility fractures in the past year. A repeat DEXA is performed and this confirms a slight decline in bone mass. Serum electrolytes including alkaline phosphatase, calcium, celiac antibodies, PTH, and 25-vitamin D levels are all normal.

How would you manage this patient?

Yousaf Ali, *Self Assessment Questions in Rheumatology,* DOI: 10.1007/ 978-1-59745-497-1,
Humana Press, a part of Springer Science + Business Media, LLC 2009

Answer: The optimal choice for this patient is an anabolic agent such as teriperatide

This patient has multiple risk factors for osteoporosis including early menopause, sex, race, and prior fracture. Assuming that she is compliant then the fact that she is fracturing despite bisphosphonate (BP) therapy indicates that she is a true BP failure.

Teriperatide has an alternative mechanism of action to BP and stimulates osteoblasts as opposed to inhibiting osteoclasts. Osteoporosis experts have developed a consensus opinion, published in the spring of 2004, to help clinicians identify appropriate patients for teriperatide therapy. Indications for its use were as follows: (1) history of vertebral fracture, T score of −3.0 or below, or age greater than 69 years, (2) fracture or unexplained bone loss in patients on antiresorptive therapy, and (3) intolerance of oral bisphosphonate therapy. Contraindications for teriparitide therapy listed include hypercalcemia, Paget's disease, a history of irradiation to the skeleton, sarcoma, or malignancy involving bone.

Miller PD, Bilezikian JP, Deal C, et al. Clinical use of teriperatide in the real world: initial insights. Endocr Pract 2004;10:139

Question 40

A 41-year-old female is referred due to 4 years of recurrent sinusitis. She has failed multiple antibiotic courses and has recently developed left-sided horizontal diplopia.

Her lab work is consistent with anemia of chronic disease and an elevated ESR of 86 mm/h. Cultures for bacteria, fungi, and tubercles are negative. A CT scan of the sinuses confirms destructive pansinusitis with a nasopharyngeal mass. Serologies are consistent with a +p-ANCA, −cANCA, and −Pr3/MPO antibody. Renal and pulmonary functions are preserved.

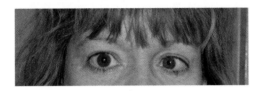

What is the differential diagnosis and most likely scenario?
What treatment is advisable?

Yousaf Ali, *Self Assessment Questions in Rheumatology,* DOI: 10.1007/ 978-1-59745-497-1,
Humana Press, a part of Springer Science + Business Media, LLC 2009

Answer: Wegener's granulomatosis (WG)

This 41-year-old patient presents with a 4-year history of recurrent sinusitis in the setting of a positive P-ANCA, destructive nasopharyngeal mass, and ophthalmoplegia.

The differential diagnosis includes infection with a refractory organism, such as mucormycosis or tuberculosis, malignancy, midline granuloma, or vasculitis. Infection and malignancy seem less likely given the chronicity and lack of positive cultures.

Although most patients with WG have antibodies to proteinase-3 and positive c-ANCA antibodies, a small minority have antibodies to p-ANCA.

This patient's inflammation has extended into the sinuses and cavernous sinus causing cranial neuropathy and ophthalmoplegia.

Optimal treatment involves oral corticosteroids and oral daily cyclophosphamide. Prior to the introduction of cytotoxic drugs this was a disease of very high mortality.

Bosch X, Guilabert A, Font J. Antineutrophil cytoplasmic antibodies. Lancet. 2006 Jul 29;368(9533):404–18. Review.

Erickson VR, Hwang PH. Wegener's granulomatosis: current trends in diagnosis and management. Curr Opin Otolaryngol Head Neck Surg. 2007 Jun;15(3):170–6. Review.

Foster WP, Greene JS, Millman B. Wegener's granulomatosis presenting as ophthalmoplegia and optic neuropathy. Otolaryngol Head Neck Surg. 1995 Jun;112(6):758–62.

Question 41

A 67-year-old diabetic African American male is referred for evaluation of chronic right ankle pain. There is a distant history of trauma and poorly controlled diabetes. He denies podagra, and serum uric acid is normal. On examination he has fair peripheral circulation, pes planus with mild ankle tenderness at the tibiotalar joint, and glove and stocking neuropathy is present. His radiograph shows diffuse demineralization and Lisfranc dislocation of the midtarsus. The joint is tapped and hemarthrosisis noted.

What is the most likely diagnosis?
Who was Lisfranc?

Yousaf Ali, *Self Assessment Questions in Rheumatology,* DOI: 10.1007/ 978-1-59745-497-1,
Humana Press, a part of Springer Science+Business Media, LLC 2009

Answer: Charcot joint

This patient has a classic Charcot joint, which is characterized by damage secondary to loss of sensation that occurs due to the patient's underlying diabetes. The features of a Charcot joint include fragmentation of bone, progressive destruction, and disorganization. Although there are many causes, diabetic neuropathy is the commonest cause in the western world. Lisfranc dislocation implies disruption of the joint between the rigid midfoot and more supple weight-bearing forefoot. Arthrocentesis frequently yields a hemarthrosis.

Lisfranc was Napolean's surgeon who described a technique to amputate the forefoot in soldiers suffering from frostbite.

Tomas MB, Patel M, Marwin SE, Palestro CJ. The diabetic foot. Br J Radiol. 2000 Apr;73(868):443–50. Review.

Question 42

A 58-year-old female from the Dominican Republic with seropositive RA of 20-year duration is seen due to fever, dyspnea, and malaise. She commenced anti-TNF therapy 1 month prior to her presentation due to poorly controlled RA. Her current medications include methotrexate, folate, celecoxib, and infliximab. Her examination shows a low-grade temperature of 100.5°F. She has chronic synovitis of the mcp/pip and wrist joints with bibasilar end inspiratory crepitations on pulmonary examination. Serum and urine microbiologic studies are negative. A CXR reveals chronic bibasilar fibrosis and a new apical infiltrate.

What is the major clinical concern in this patient?

Yousaf Ali, *Self Assessment Questions in Rheumatology,* DOI: 10.1007/ 978-1-59745-497-1,
Humana Press, a part of Springer Science+Business Media, LLC 2009

Answer: Tuberculosis (TB)

This patient has developed a new apical infiltrate in the setting of anti-TNF therapy. TNF is a pleiotropic molecule important in immune surveillance and host defense. It is also important in granuloma formation and maintenance. TNF-deficient knock-out mice develop fatal TB and listeriosis. Reactivation of TB is a well-recognized complication of anti-TNF therapy, and patients should be screened with skin testing prior to initiation of therapy.

Crum NF, Lederman ER, Wallace MR. Infections associated with tumor necrosis factor-alpha antagonists. Medicine. 2005 Sep;84(5):291–302. Review.

Flynn JL, Goldstein MM, Chan J, Triebold KJ, Pfeffer K, Lowenstein CJ, Schreiber R, Mak TW, Bloom BR. Tumor necrosis factor-α is required in the protective immune response against *Mycobacterium tuberculosis* in mice. Immunity 1995;2:561–72.

Hamilton CD. Tuberculosis in the cytokine era: what rheumatologists need to know. Arthritis Rheum. 2003 Aug;48(8):2085–91. Review.

Question 43

You are asked to see a 46-year-old alcoholic male to help with the management of presumed gout. He presented with acute bilateral ankle pain and swelling. He has chronic low back stiffness. The admitting physician has performed arthrocentesis of the ankle joint, which confirmed type 2 inflammatory fluid without crystals. Lab work reveals intact hematologic and renal function and UA = 8.4 mg/dl.

On examination he has bilateral tenderness over the right metatarsal heads, thickening of the Achilles tendon with exquisite tenderness, and warm bilateral ankle effusions. Radiographs of the spine confirm right sacroiliac fusion. He is treated with colchicine without any improvement.

What is the most likely diagnosis?
What else would you look for on examination?

Yousaf Ali, *Self Assessment Questions in Rheumatology,* DOI: 10.1007/ 978-1-59745-497-1,
Humana Press, a part of Springer Science + Business Media, LLC 2009

Answer: Ankylosing spondylitis (AS)

This 46-year-old male presents with axial stiffness, metatarsal inflammation, enthesopathy, and sacroiliitis. This is highly suggestive of a reactive arthritis or AS. Gout has been effectively excluded by the absence of urate crystals and would not typically present with Achilles tendonitis or sacroiliitis.

Other things to examine for would be digital pitting, psoriatic plaques, stigmata of inflammatory bowel disease, urogenital infection, or uveitis. The elevated uric acid is of no clinical significance and the colchicine should be stopped.

Reveille JD, Arnett FC. Spondyloarthritis: update on pathogenesis and management. Am J Med. 2005 Jun;118(6):592–603. Review.

Question 44

A 27-year-old female with SLE is referred with new onset pleuritic chest pain. She has a history of arthritis and mucositis, which has been controlled on NSAIDs and antimalarial agents. She has a history of two second trimester miscarriages.

On examination she has sinus tachycardia, RV heave, and a loud P2. Diffuse livedo reticularis is noted. Lung examination is clear and CXR appears normal apart from slightly oligemic fields. She is mildly hypoxic and is using accessory muscles of respiration.

What is the most likely diagnosis?

Yousaf Ali, *Self Assessment Questions in Rheumatology,* DOI: 10.1007/ 978-1-59745-497-1,
Humana Press, a part of Springer Science+Business Media, LLC 2009

Answer: Pulmonary embolus

This patient with SLE most likely has antiphospholipid syndrome (APS) with a history of recurrent pregnancy loss and livedo reticularis. Her examination reveals elevated right-sided pulmonary pressure consistent with right ventricular strain. Pericarditis should also be considered although it would be less likely given the physical findings. APS is a disease of recurrent vascular thrombosis and fetal loss associated with antibodies to membrane phospholipids. Approximately 40% of patients with SLE have anticardiolipin antibodies but only 10% have APS syndrome.

Lockshin MD. Update on antiphospholipid syndrome. Bull NYU Hosp Jt Dis. 2006;64(1–2):57–59.

Question 45

A 78-year-old female is admitted with malaise, fever to 101°F and unintentional weight loss. She has a 45-year history of seropositive erosive RA controlled on methotrexate and more recently intravenous anti-TNF therapy. She has known interstitial lung disease. On examination she is cachectic, with chronic deformities and low-grade synovitis. Her lung examination reveals coarse bibasilar crepitations. She has axillary lymphadenopathy and bipedal edema. Lab work reveals a normocytic anemia, mild eosinophilia, and hypoalbuminemia but otherwise intact renal and hepatic function. Urinalysis is benign.

Viral, rickettsial, and microbiologic studies are normal; a CT scan reveals marked hilar lymphadenopathy and chronic fibrotic changes at the lung bases. A tuberculin skin test is negative.

What is the most likely diagnosis?

Yousaf Ali, *Self Assessment Questions in Rheumatology,* DOI: 10.1007/ 978-1-59745-497-1,
Humana Press, a part of Springer Science+Business Media, LLC 2009

Answer: Lymphoma

This patient with chronic RA presents with fever, lymphadenopathy, eosinophilia, and weight loss in the setting of a negative infectious disease evaluation. The differential diagnosis includes infection, TB, and lymphoma. The latter diagnosis is most likely given the negative microbiologic studies.

Patients with chronic RA are predisposed to lymphoma, and although not clear, in 2007 this risk might be further amplified by concomitant anti-TNF therapy. Patients with the most severe disease activity scores have the greatest risk of developing lymphomas.

When using biologic agents the benefits of treatment must be weighed against potential toxicity.

Franklin J, Lunt M, Bunn D, Symmons D, Silman A. Incidence of lymphoma in a large primary care derived cohort of cases of inflammatory polyarthritis. Ann Rheum Dis. 2006;65:617–22.

Wolfe F, Michaud K. Lymphoma in rheumatoid arthritis: the effect of methotrexate and anti-tumor necrosis factor therapy in 18,572 patients. Arthritis Rheum. 2004 Jun;50(6):1740–51.

Question 46

A 46-year-old male immigrant is admitted for further evaluation of a pulmonary artery aneurysm noted on an incidental CXR. He has a prior history of uveitis and arthritis. On examination there is hypophyon, erythema nodosum, and oral ulceration.

What is the most likely diagnosis?

Yousaf Ali, *Self Assessment Questions in Rheumatology,* DOI: 10.1007/ 978-1-59745-497-1,
Humana Press, a part of Springer Science + Business Media, LLC 2009

Answer: Behcet's syndrome

This patient has classic Behcet's syndrome (BS), which is an HLA-B51-associated disease characterized by recurrent orogenital ulceration, thrombophlebitis, uveitis, and vasculitis. Skin lesions include erythema nodosum, abnormal pathergy, and folliculitis.

The etiology is unknown but this is a disease with racial preference along the old Silk route from the Mediterranean to China. Pulmonary artery aneurysms are a rare cause of pulmonary hemorrhage and should raise the suspicion of BS.

Alpagut U, Ugurlucan M, Dayioglu E. Major arterial involvement and review of Behcet's disease. Ann Vasc Surg. 2007 Mar;21(2):232–39. Review.

Uzun O, Akpolat T, Erkan L. Pulmonary vasculitis in Behcet disease: a cumulative analysis. Chest. 2005 Jun;127(6):2243–53. Review.

Yazici H, Fresko I, Yurdakul S. Behçet's syndrome: disease manifestations, management, and advances in treatment. Nat Clin Pract Rheumatol. 2007 Mar;3(3):148–55. Review.

Question 47

A 67-year-old African American female with dialysis-dependent renal failure is evaluated for recurrent carpal tunnel syndrome. She has had two injections in the past 6 months, which were of temporary benefit. On examination she has atrophy of the thenar eminens and weakness of opponens muscles. Phalen's sign is positive and her grip is diminished.

What complication has occurred?

Yousaf Ali, *Self Assessment Questions in Rheumatology,* DOI: 10.1007/ 978-1-59745-497-1,
Humana Press, a part of Springer Science + Business Media, LLC 2009

Answer: B2 Amyloid.

Dialysis-related amyloidosis (DRA) is a complication of end-stage renal disease that results from retention of beta2-microglobulin (beta2M) and its deposition as amyloid fibrils into osteoarticular tissue. The clinical manifestations usually develop after several years of dialysis dependence and include carpal tunnel syndrome, destructive arthropathy, bone cysts, and fractures. Risk factors for the development of DRA include age, duration of dialysis treatment, use of low-flux dialysis membrane, use of low-purity dialysate, monocyte chemoattractant protein-1 GG genotype, and apolipoprotein E4 allele.

Surgical management is usually successful but can result in recurrence. An extended release procedure may be more successful.

Dember LM, Jaber BL.Dialysis-related amyloidosis: late finding or hidden epidemic? Semin Dial. 2006 Mar/Apr;19(2):105–9. Review.

Wilson SW, Pollard RE, Lees VC. Management of carpal tunnel syndrome in renal dialysis patients using an extended carpal tunnel release procedure. J Plast Reconstr Aesthet Surg. 2008 Sep;61(9):1090–4.

Question 48

A 55-year-old female with chronic renal failure is seen for evaluation of lower extremity edema and ankle pain. One month before she had an MRI with gadolinium for low back pain. On examination a woody induration is noted over the shins bilaterally. A skin biopsy is performed, which reveals mucin deposition and a proliferation of fibroblasts and elastic fibers.

What is the most likely diagnosis? Discuss.

Yousaf Ali, *Self Assessment Questions in Rheumatology*, DOI: 10.1007/ 978-1-59745-497-1,
Humana Press, a part of Springer Science + Business Media, LLC 2009

Answer: Nephrogenic fibrosing dermopathy

Nephrogenic fibrosing dermopathy/nephrogenic systemic fibrosis (NSF) is an emerging scleromyxedema-like cutaneous disorder of unknown cause that is seen in patients with renal failure; the number of reported cases has grown significantly since its first recognition. Virtually all cases of NSF have been associated with the administration of gadolinium-containing contrast media. Skin biopsies of affected areas reveal thickened collagen bundles, mucin deposition, and proliferation of fibroblasts and elastic fibers. The etiology is unknown but gadolinium may act as a stimulant to attract circulating fibrocytes to the dermis. Ideally gadolinium should be avoided unless absolutely necessary in patients with renal failure.

Peak AS, Sheller A. Risk factors for developing gadolinium-induced nephrogenic systemic fibrosis. Ann Pharmacother. 2007 Sep;41(9):1481–5. Review.

Solomon GJ, Rosen PP, Wu E. The role of gadolinium in triggering nephrogenic systemic fibrosis/nephrogenic fibrosing dermopathy. Arch Pathol Lab Med. 2007 Oct;131(10):1515–16. Review.

Question 49

You are asked to see a patient with refractory erythema nodosum. He is a 46-year-old ex-intravenous drug abuser who has had painful raised lesions over his shins for 4 months. He also complains of low-grade fever, arthralgia, and abdominal pain. He has lost 15 lbs in 6 months. On examination temperature is 38.3°C, and there is evidence of clubbing and tender raised nodules over the anterior shins. His cardiac examination reveals a 3/6 ejection systolic murmur at the right sternal border and 2/6 early diastolic murmur. BP = 166/64. Pulmonary examination is normal, and abdominal examination reveals tenderness in the RUQ. A CXR is normal.

What diagnostic test should be performed?

Yousaf Ali, *Self Assessment Questions in Rheumatology,* DOI: 10.1007/ 978-1-59745-497-1,
Humana Press, a part of Springer Science+Business Media, LLC 2009

Answer: Blood cultures

This patient has endocarditis with valvular insufficiency and probable streptococcal bacteremia. Streptococcus is a common cause of erythema nodosum (EN). Other causes include sarcoidosis, TB, yersinia, fungal infections, inflammatory bowel disease, Behcet's disease, and drugs such as sulfonamides.

Mert A, Kumbasar H, Ozaras R, Erten S, Tasli L, Tabak F, Ozturk R. Erythema nodosum: an evaluation of 100 cases. Clin Exp Rheumatol. 2007 Jul/Aug;25(4):563–70.

Mert A, Ozaras R, Tabak F, Pekmezci S, Demirkesen C, Ozturk R. Erythema nodosum: an experience of 10 years. Scand J Infect Dis. 2004;36(6–7):424–7.

Question 50

A 29-year-old resident is seen for refractory foot pain of 1-week duration. Her past medical history is significant for anorexia nervosa for which she attends monthly counseling classes. Her weight is 87 lbs, height 5'6". On examination she has diffuse tenderness at the midfoot. She denies trauma or swelling.

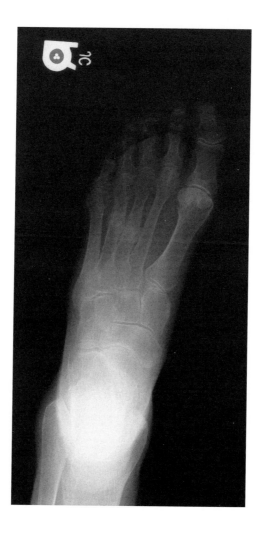

What is the diagnosis?

Yousaf Ali, *Self Assessment Questions in Rheumatology*, DOI: 10.1007/ 978-1-59745-497-1, Humana Press, a part of Springer Science + Business Media, LLC 2009

Answer: Metatarsal fracture

Because of anorexia nervosa and low body mass this patient is at a higher risk for osteoporosis and fragility fracture. This radiograph clearly shows two healing metatarsal fractures, which are the cause of the patient's pain. The decreased bone density in patients with anorexia nervosa (AN) is due to the many effects on bone metabolism of amenorrhea, reduced levels of insulin-like growth factor-1 (IGF-1), high cortisol levels, and weight loss. Although bisphosphonates have been used the most effective treatment involves resumption of menses and weight restoration.

Do Carmo I, Mascarenhas M, Macedo A, Silva A, Santos I, Bouça D, Myatt J, Sampaio D. A study of bone density change in patients with anorexia nervosa. Eur Eat Disord Rev. 2007 Nov;15(6):457–62.

Wolfert A, Mehler PS. Osteoporosis: prevention and treatment in anorexia nervosa. Eat Weight Disord. 2002 Jun;7(2):72–81. Review.

Question 51

A 59-year-old diabetic male has pain over the anterior hip and groin. He has recently had angina and has started a vigorous exercise regimen. On examination there is clicking of the hip with flexion but no pain with rotation. Distal neurovascular examination is intact. A radiograph of the right hip and pelvis is normal.

What is the most likely diagnosis?
How would you treat him?

Yousaf Ali, *Self Assessment Questions in Rheumatology,* DOI: 10.1007/ 978-1-59745-497-1,
Humana Press, a part of Springer Science+Business Media, LLC 2009

Answer: Iliopsoas bursitis

The iliopsoas muscle passes anterior to the pelvic brim and hip capsule in a groove between the anterior inferior iliac spine laterally and iliopectineal eminence medially. It acts as one of the hip flexors and is occasionally injured in excessive hip flexion or trauma. Patients often have an insidious onset of anterior thigh pain, which often radiates down to the knee and is associated with hip clicking.

Treatment involves physical therapy to alleviate pain, spasm, and swelling.

Johnston CA, Wiley JP, Lindsay DM, Wiseman DA. Iliopsoas bursitis and tendinitis. A review. Sports Med. 1998 Apr;25(4):271–83. Review.

Question 52

A 35-year-old markedly obese female is referred for evaluation of scleroderma. She is asymptomatic but has limited sclerodactly and skin thickening of the face, digits. Nailfold examination shows dilated capillary loops. Lab and urine data are normal. She is diagnosed with CREST syndrome on the basis of esophageal dysfunction and Raynauds.

Cardiac examination reveals a normal S2, and pulmonary examination is clear without rales.

A baseline 2D ECHO reveals a PA pressure of 45 mmHg (nl < 25) but PFTs and DLCO are normal.

What is the next appropriate step?

Yousaf Ali, *Self Assessment Questions in Rheumatology,* DOI: 10.1007/ 978-1-59745-497-1, Humana Press, a part of Springer Science + Business Media, LLC 2009

Answer: Observation with repeat ECHO in 4–6 months

This patient has CREST syndrome and elevated right-sided pulmonary pressures by conventional 2D echocardiogram. Since pulmonary hypertension is a major cause of mortality in these patients, further investigations are warranted. Her Echocardiogram reveals pulmonary hypertension (normal mean PA pressure<25 mmHg) although there is a clear disconnect between her symptoms, examination, and the echo findings. There are differing opinions in this scenario but in an asymptomatic patient she could probably be observed for clinical deterioration or symptoms. A 6-min walk test is also helpful and if abnormal, a right heart catheterization can be considered. This patient had normal PA pressures on right heart catheterization. This case illustrates the limitations of accuracy of echocardiography in obese patients.

Denton CP, Cailes JB, Phillips GD, Wells AU, Black CM, Bois RM. Comparison of Doppler echocardiography and right heart catheterization to assess pulmonary hypertension in systemic sclerosis. Br J Rheumatol. 1997 Feb;36(2):239–43.

Gurubhagavatula I, Palevsky HI. Pulmonary hypertension in systemic autoimmune disease. Rheum Dis Clin North Am. 1997;23:365–94.

Question 53

A 28-year-old female with SLE is diagnosed with class 4 nephritis. She is started on immunosuppressive therapy with pulse cyclophosphamide, prednisone, and furosemide.

Three months after the initial presentation she is admitted with hypertension and has a witnessed tonic clonic seizure in the ER. Her BP is 190/115 and she appears post ictal when you examine her. There is no rash, synovitis, or evidence of serositis. An LP is unremarkable without evidence for infection or cerebritis.

A brain MRI reveals multiple hyperintensity lesions in the occipital lobe.

What complication has occurred?

Yousaf Ali, *Self Assessment Questions in Rheumatology,* DOI: 10.1007/ 978-1-59745-497-1,
Humana Press, a part of Springer Science + Business Media, LLC 2009

Answer: Posterior reversible encephalopathy syndrome

Posterior reversible encephalopathy syndrome (PRES) or reversible posterior leu-koencephalopathy syndrome (RPLS) is an increasingly recognized neurologic disor-der with characteristic computed tomographic (CT) and magnetic resonance (MR) imaging findings, and is associated with a multitude of diverse clinical entities. These include acute glomerulonephritis, preeclampsia and eclampsia, systemic lupus ery-thematosus, thrombotic thrombocytopenic purpura, and hemolytic-uremic syndrome, as well as drug toxicity from agents such as cyclosporine, tacrolimus, cisplatin, and erythropoietin. Most, but not all, cases manifest with acute to subacute hypertension, and seizures are also frequent. Two pathophysiologic mechanisms for PRES have been proposed. One postulates cerebral vasospasm with resulting ischemia within the involved territories, whereas the other posits a breakdown in cerebrovascular autoreg-ulation with ensuing interstitial extravasation of fluid.

This case is particularly difficult in that a patient with SLE who presents with a seizure and hypertension has to be excluded for active cerebritis or nephritis. The normal lumbar puncture and characteristic MRI findings are highly suggestive of PRES. Treatment involves normalization of BP, removing offending agents such as cytoxan, and prevention of further seizures.

Kur JK, Esdaile JM. Posterior reversible encephalopathy syndrome – an underrecognized mani-festation of systemic lupus erythematosus. J Rheumatol. 2006 Nov;33(11):2178–83. Review.

Ishimori ML, Pressman BD, Wallace DJ, Weisman MH. Posterior reversible encephalopathy syndrome: another manifestation of CNS SLE? Lupus. 2007;16(6):436–43. Review.

Question 54

A 25-year-old female has had low back pain for 6 months. She has an unremarkable past history apart from one prior episode of uveitis. Review of systems is negative for diarrhea, urethral discharge/travel, or constitutional symptoms. Her examination reveals a positive FABER sign and tenderness over the lower lumbosacral spine and sacroiliac joint.

The rest of the joint and skin examination is normal apart from subungual hyperkeratosis and oil spots.

What is the most likely diagnosis?

Yousaf Ali, *Self Assessment Questions in Rheumatology,* DOI: 10.1007/ 978-1-59745-497-1,
Humana Press, a part of Springer Science + Business Media, LLC 2009

Answer: Psoriatic arthritis (PsA)

Cutaneous manifestations of psoriasis include oil spots or "oil droplets" – orange-brown patches seen through the nail plate, nail pitting, onycholysis, and subungual hyperkeratosis. Psoriatic nail disease is often associated with psoriatic arthropathy. This patient also has evidence of inflammatory low back pain, uveitis,and sacroiliitis, which are all characteristic of PsA. FABER's test (flexion, abduction, external rotation) is a test for the sacroiliac joint and hip disease. If the patient has pain in the groin it suggests hip pathology but if the pain is in the sacroiliac area it is more consistent with sacroiliitis.

Paiva ES, Macaluso DC, Edwards A, Rosenbaum JT. Characterisation of uveitis in patients with psoriatic arthritis. Ann Rheum Dis. 2000 Jan;59(1):67–70.

Turkiewicz AM, Moreland LW. Psoriatic arthritis: current concepts on pathogenesis-oriented therapeutic options. Arthritis Rheum. 2007 Apr;56(4):1051–66. Review.

Zeboulon N, Dougados M, Gossec L. Prevalence and characteristics of uveitis in spondylarthropathies: a systematic literature review. Ann Rheum Dis. 2008;67:955–9.

Question 55

A 67-year-old Caucasian female is referred for left forearm pain for 2 months duration. She describes pain that only occurs with activity. Her PMH includes newly diagnosed PMR, CAD, and spinal stenosis. Her current medications include prednisone 5 mg daily, aspirin, and atenolol. On examination she is mildly cushingoid with an absent left radial pulse. There is no peripheral synovitis, and examination of the forearm and elbow joint is unremarkable. Resisted extension of the wrist fails to reproduce the pain. There is a faint left subclavian bruit.

Her laboratory data reveal an elevated ESR of 80 mm/h, and normal renal and biochemical parameters. She has a mild normocytic anemia.

What is the most likely scenario?
What is the next best step to evaluate this?

Yousaf Ali, *Self Assessment Questions in Rheumatology,* DOI: 10.1007/ 978-1-59745-497-1,
Humana Press, a part of Springer Science + Business Media, LLC 2009

Answer: Large vessel vasculitis

This patient has a recent diagnosis of PMR and now presents with claudication of the left upper extremity in the setting of an absent pulse and markedly elevated inflammatory markers. At this point the diagnosis of exclusion is temporal arteritis (TA) with large vessel involvement. The presence of a subclavian bruit also suggests proximal occlusion. Takayasu's arteritis is also a possibility but less likely given the patient's age and ethnicity. Atherosclerosis needs to be considered but again should not be associated with this degree of inflammation. Large-vessel involvement in giant cell arteritis occurs in over a quarter of patients with this disease. Stenosis of the primary and secondary branches of the aorta may cause claudication and tissue gangrene, whereas aortitis may lead to aneurysm formation and dissection, often many years after the initial diagnosis. The important thing here is to treat the inflammation and ensure that no other organs are involved. A temporal artery biopsy is the best next step. Occasionally TA can be silent and only becomes apparent when a biopsy is performed.

Bongartz T, Matteson EL. Large-vessel involvement in giant cell arteritis. Curr Opin Rheumatol. 2006 Jan;18(1):10–17. Review.

Kwon CM, Hong YH, Chun KA, Cho IH, Kim MJ, Shin DG, Hyun MS, Kim YJ. A case of silent giant cell arteritis involving the entire aorta, carotid artery, and brachial artery screened by integrated PET/CT. Clin Rheumatol. 2007 Nov;26(11):1959–62.

Radiology Section

Question

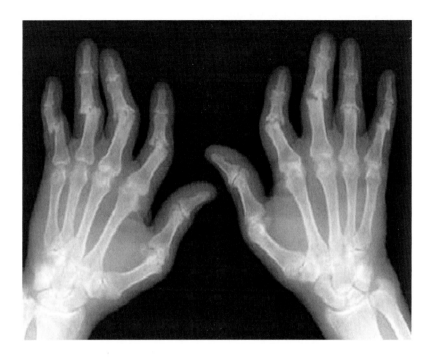

What is the diagnosis?

Yousaf Ali, *Self Assessment Questions in Rheumatology,* DOI: 10.1007/ 978-1-59745-497-1,
Humana Press, a part of Springer Science+Business Media, LLC 2009

Answer: Psoriatic arthritis with arthritis mutilans

This is a very destructive form of psoriatic arthritis with significant periarticular bone resorption. The erosions can cause a "pencil in cup" deformity where one articular surface is eroded creating a pointed appearance; the articulating bone can be concave, resembling an upside down cup.

Question 57

This patient has severe hip pain.

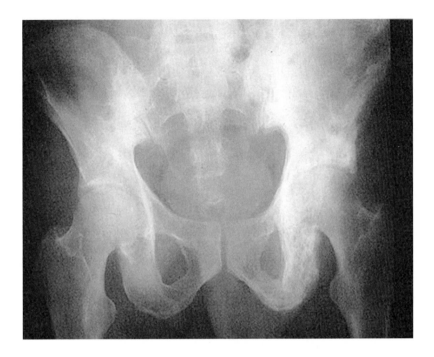

What does the X-ray show and what advice would you give to the orthopaedic surgeon?

Yousaf Ali, *Self Assessment Questions in Rheumatology,* DOI: 10.1007/ 978-1-59745-497-1,
Humana Press, a part of Springer Science + Business Media, LLC 2009

Answer: Paget's disease

Diffuse involvement of the left hemipelvis is manifested by areas of mixed sclerosis and lucency. There is also involvement of the right hemipelvis near the right sacro-iliac joint, secondary hip osteoarthritis, and thickening of the iliopectineal line.

Antiresorptive treatment should be commenced prior to hip replacement to decrease the hypervascularity and decrease the risk of perioperative bleeding.

Question 58

This patient has postpartum pain.

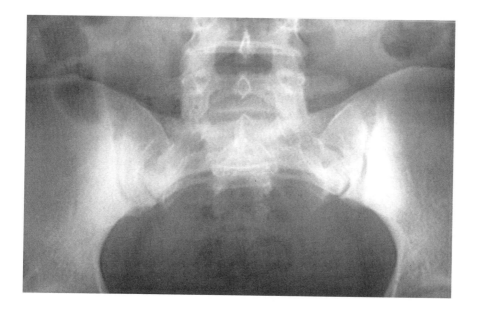

What does the X-ray show?

Yousaf Ali, *Self Assessment Questions in Rheumatology,* DOI: 10.1007/ 978-1-59745-497-1,
Humana Press, a part of Springer Science + Business Media, LLC 2009

Answer: Osteitis condensans ilii

Osteitis condensans ilii (OCI) is the radiologic appearance of increased sclerosis in the inferior aspect of the body of the iliac bone arising in a triangular configuration from the lateral aspect of the sacroiliac joint (SI). It is seen most commonly in multiparous women, but also in some degenerative conditions. It is merely a benign reflection of bone remodeling with response to stress, but with the increased radiologic density it is indicative of sclerosis. The SI joints themselves are normal or may feature some degenerative – but not inflammatory or erosive – changes. This condition may sometimes be confused with sacroiliitis, but it can be differentiated by its unilateral nature, lack of erosive or other inflammatory features, both locally and in the spine, and the general absence of clinical symptoms.

Question 59

This patient has refractory wrist pain.

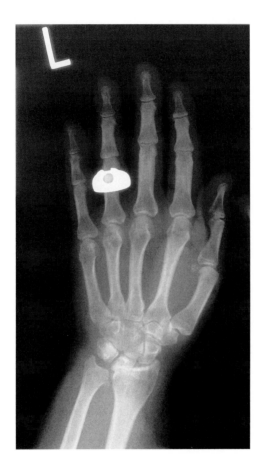

What is the diagnosis and what does the radiograph show?

Yousaf Ali, *Self Assessment Questions in Rheumatology,* DOI: 10.1007/ 978-1-59745-497-1,
Humana Press, a part of Springer Science + Business Media, LLC 2009

Answer: Kienbock's disease: avascular necrosis of the lunate

Kienbock's disease is breakdown of the lunate bone, a carpal bone in the wrist that articulates with the radius in the forearm. Fragmentation and collapse of the lunate occurs and has classically been attributed to arterial disruption, but may also occur after events that produce venous congestion with elevated interosseous pressure.

Question 60

A 60-year male is evaluated with a history of spinal cord injury and knee pain.

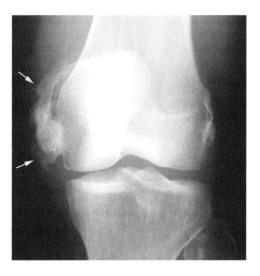

What does the X-ray show?

Yousaf Ali, *Self Assessment Questions in Rheumatology,* DOI: 10.1007/ 978-1-59745-497-1,
Humana Press, a part of Springer Science + Business Media, LLC 2009

Answer: Heteretopic ossification

Heterotopic ossification (HO) is the abnormal formation of true bone within extraskeletal soft tissues. The etiology is unclear but this condition can complicate bone forming disorders, joint replacement, blunt trauma, and spinal cord injury.

Question 61

A 55-year-old male has refractory low back pain alleviated by swimming.

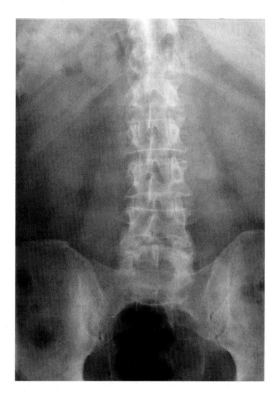

What does the pelvic film show?

Yousaf Ali, *Self Assessment Questions in Rheumatology,* DOI: 10.1007/ 978-1-59745-497-1,
Humana Press, a part of Springer Science + Business Media, LLC 2009

Answer: Right sacroiliac fusion consistent with a spondyloarthropathy

Question 62

A 32-year-old male weightlifter has right shoulder pain.

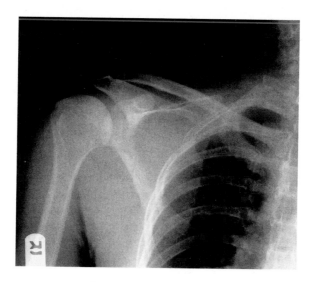

What does the X-ray show?

Yousaf Ali, *Self Assessment Questions in Rheumatology,* DOI: 10.1007/ 978-1-59745-497-1,
Humana Press, a part of Springer Science + Business Media, LLC 2009

Answer: Right distal clavicle osteolysis induced by weightlifting

Question 63

This patient with chronic renal failure had a recent MRI with contrast.

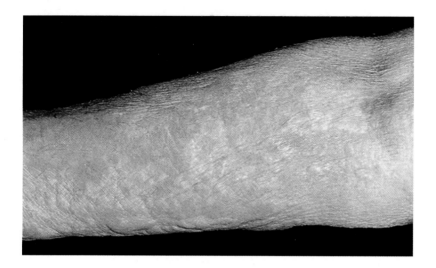

What complication has occurred?

Yousaf Ali, *Self Assessment Questions in Rheumatology,* DOI: 10.1007/ 978-1-59745-497-1,
Humana Press, a part of Springer Science + Business Media, LLC 2009

Answer: Nephrogenic fibrosing dermopathy

This is a rare complication of gadolinium that occurs primarily in people with renal failure. See Q48.

Question 64

This elderly female has osteoporosis and new pelvic pain.

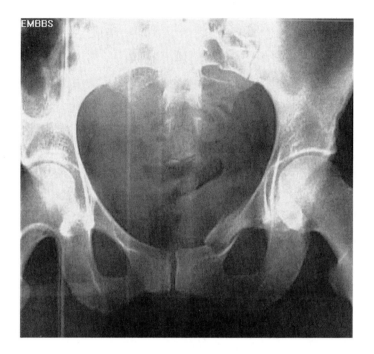

What is the diagnosis?

Yousaf Ali, *Self Assessment Questions in Rheumatology,* DOI: 10.1007/ 978-1-59745-497-1,
Humana Press, a part of Springer Science + Business Media, LLC 2009

Answer: Insufficiency fracture of the superior pubic ramus

Question 65

This 45-year-old male has 5 years of RA controlled on plaquenil.

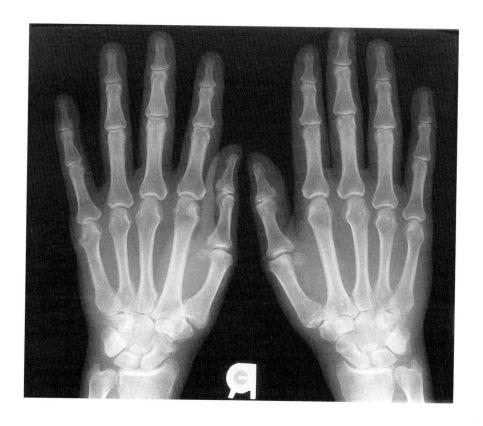

What does his X-ray show?
What would you advise him?

Yousaf Ali, *Self Assessment Questions in Rheumatology,* DOI: 10.1007/ 978-1-59745-497-1,
Humana Press, a part of Springer Science+Business Media, LLC 2009

Answer: An erosion at the right fifth MCP joint

A discussion should be had about more aggressive remittive therapy.

Question 66

This elderly female has sudden onset of excruciating shoulder pain.

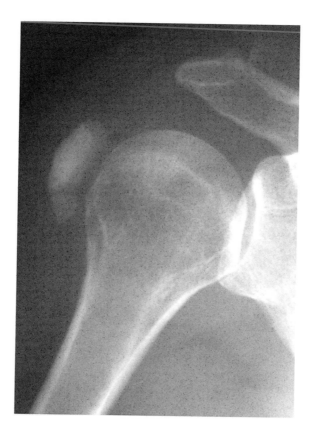

What is the Diagnosis?

Yousaf Ali, *Self Assessment Questions in Rheumatology,* DOI: 10.1007/ 978-1-59745-497-1,
Humana Press, a part of Springer Science+Business Media, LLC 2009

Answer: Calcific tendonitis

This is a disorder characterized by deposits of hydroxyapatite (a crystalline calcium phosphate) in any tendon of the body, but most commonly in the tendons of the rotator cuff (shoulder), causing pain and inflammation.

Question 67

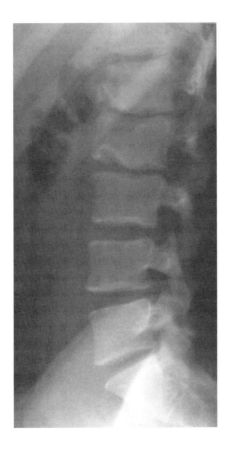

Describe this X-ray.

Yousaf Ali, *Self Assessment Questions in Rheumatology,* DOI: 10.1007/ 978-1-59745-497-1,
Humana Press, a part of Springer Science+Business Media, LLC 2009

Answer: Schmorl's node at L2

Schmorl's nodes are defined as herniations of the intervertebral disc through the vertebral end-plate. Schmorl's nodes are common, especially with minor degeneration of the aging spine. Schmorl's nodes usually cause no symptoms, but reflect that *wear and tear* of the spine has occurred over time. This radiograph also shows a defect at the anterior body of L1 reflecting protrusion of the intervertebral disk beneath the ring apophysis of the growing vertebral body.

Question 68

This 77-year-old male is asymptomatic. A routine chest radiograph notes an abnormality in the spine. His lab work is normal.

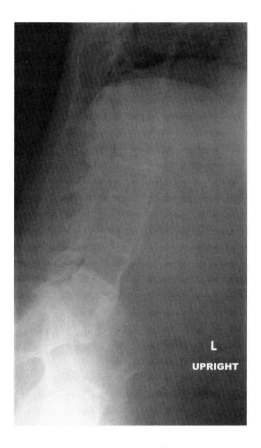

What is the most likely diagnosis based on this lateral view?
What other film would be helpful?
How would you manage him?

Yousaf Ali, *Self Assessment Questions in Rheumatology,* DOI: 10.1007/ 978-1-59745-497-1,
Humana Press, a part of Springer Science + Business Media, LLC 2009

Answer: Diffuse skeletal hyperostosis (DISH) syndrome

A pelvic/ sacroiliac view would be helpful to exclude sacroiliitis. AS is very unlikely at this age. See Q18.

No treatment is indicated.

Question 69

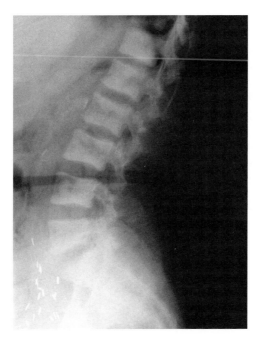

Describe these X-rays.
What is the diagnosis?

Yousaf Ali, *Self Assessment Questions in Rheumatology,* DOI: 10.1007/ 978-1-59745-497-1,
Humana Press, a part of Springer Science + Business Media, LLC 2009

Answer: Renal osteodystrophy with Rugger jersey spine. Note the renal transplant.

Renal osteodystrophy combines features of secondary hyperparathyroidism, rickets, osteomalacia, and osteoporosis. Bone resorption in renal osteodystrophy is quite complex. Renal retention of phosphate results in hyperphosphatemia, which reduces serum ionized calcium levels, therefore inducing hyperparathyroidism. The hyperparathyroidism increases bone resorption, which may normalize serum calcium levels by releasing the osseous storage of calcium. The various sites of bone resorption include the subperiosteal region of the phalanges, the phalangeal tufts, proximal femur, proximal tibia, proximal humerus, distal clavicle, and calvarial trabeculae. If parathormone levels are mildly elevated over a longer period of time, its effect on bone tends to be anabolic. These effects include excessive maturation of osteoblasts leading to new bone formation and increased laying down of osteoid, which calcifies under the influence of secondarily elevated serum calcium levels. This patient has classic endplate involvement, which results in the appearance of a "Rugger jersey."

Question 70

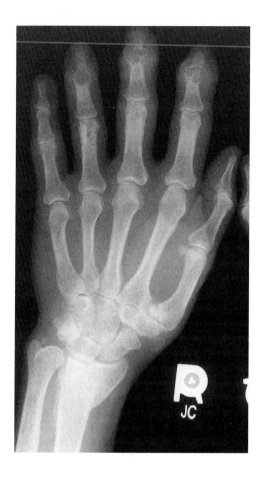

Describe the X-ray.
What is the diagnosis?

Yousaf Ali, *Self Assessment Questions in Rheumatology,* DOI: 10.1007/ 978-1-59745-497-1,
Humana Press, a part of Springer Science + Business Media, LLC 2009

Answer: Gout with erosions

Characteristic radiographic findings of gout are well-defined, punched-out erosions with overhanging edges, preservation of the joint space, lack of periarticular osteopenia, asymmetrical involvement, soft tissue nodules, and intraosseous calcifications.

Index